Vintage Hairstyles

Vintage Hairstyles

SIMPLE STEPS FOR RETRO
HAIR WITH A MODERN TWIST

EMMA SUNDH
SARAH WING
PHOTOGRAPHS BY MARTINA ANKARFYR

CHRONICLE BOOKS
SAN FRANCISCO

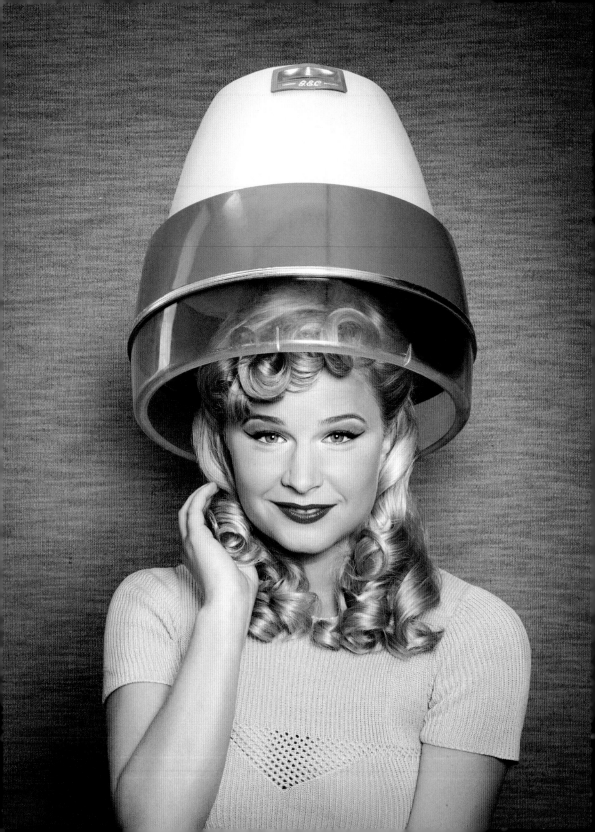

Contents

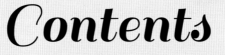

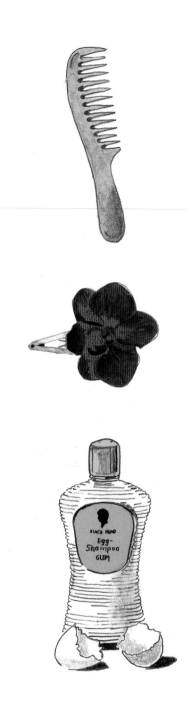

INTRODUCTION

Have you dreamed of getting retro hair in a flash? You've come to the right place, darling. Welcome to *Vintage Hairstyles*.

Forget hood dryers and hours of trying to get every little curl in place, which only leads to sore arms. I've spent hours perfecting hairstyles using retro techniques, which has inspired me to modernize and simplify the world's oldest accessory—the hairdo.

Some things have changed for the better since the vintage years. Today, we have access to faster techniques. We have curling irons (that don't burn your hair off), heat protectants (your hair will thank you), and my personal savior—hair spray. With the help of these innovations—and a few others—creating a vintage hairdo doesn't take any longer than styling a modern bob cut!

I've refined techniques, removed unnecessary steps, and come up with a few tricks of my own that will help you along the way. That's exactly what this book is about: easy tricks with fabulous results. Naturally, I'll also share a few old-time goodies like pin curls, finger waves, and rolls, which I treat exactly the way people did back in the day.

In making this book, I handpicked a few of my salon clients to show you that anyone can create these styles. You don't need a contract with Warner Brothers to enhance your great looks and become a femme fatale from the '40s, a bombshell from the '50s, or a vixen from the '60s. Find the inspiration in this book to create the style you've always dreamed of or to fine-tune the great look you already have.

Soon, you'll master all the tricks and techniques you need to vary your look and become your best you. The possibilities are endless.

A motto I've always cherished (and which was especially true in the 1940s) is: Great hair does wonders for any outfit. Learn to work your hair and you've got an eye-catching accessory free of charge. Wear the same dress and switch up your hair and you've got a whole new outfit!

I find inspiration for hairstyles everywhere— in old pictures of glamorous actresses and in albums found at flea markets featuring everyday girls. The feminine appeal of billowing curls and the magnificence of an artistic party updo is a visual treat, inspiring my own creativity. There's always a new shape or style to be discovered around the corner.

I have been styling hair for ten years now, and my business has always been about inspiration and innovation. In my opinion, you're free to mix new and old to create a personal style that's all your own.

Have fun curling, pinning, and rolling!

Sarah Wing

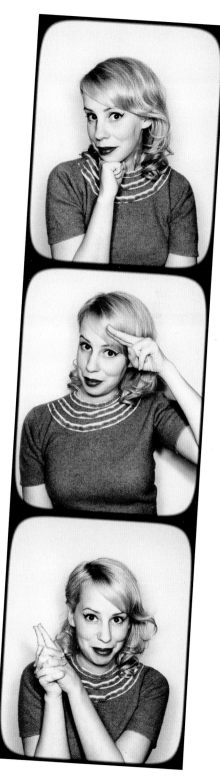

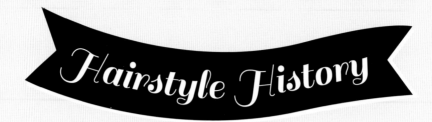

Hairstyle History

HISTORY CAN BE RETOLD THROUGH HAIR SALON VISITS.
THE 1910S SAW THE BIRTH OF THE BOB CUT, THE WARTIME
'40S INCLUDED LIPS PAINTED RED, AND THE REBELLIOUS '60S
WELCOMED THE PONYTAIL. SUPERFICIAL? FAR FROM IT.
A HAIRCUT CAN SPARK A WOMAN'S EMANCIPATION
JUST AS IT CAN EXPRESS POLITICS, ECONOMICS, AND
WOMEN'S ISSUES. HAIRSTYLES MAKE HEADLINES—
AND DID SO FROM THE 1910S TO THE 1960S.

THE 1910s

At the dawn of the twentieth century, at the very height of industrialization, things began to change. Scissors were sharpened and long hair was cut off. Until this time, hair had been gathered into large pompadours. The common practice for women had been to simply let the hair grow . . . grow . . . and grow some more. As a rule, women didn't cut their hair at all during the 1910s. There were no hair salons for women; the only thing that even came close were men's barbershops, but no women went there, since the barbershop was an exclusively male territory. Here, beards were cut and shaved with knives and the expertly waxed dandy mustaches were styled with care, at least the beards and mustaches of those who could afford it.

The emerging newly industrial society was anything but equal. Gaps between classes were huge and poverty was widespread. The outbreak of World War I in 1914 didn't help the situation. Fashion and hairstyles distinguished the rich from the poor, especially in wartime, when importing goods like fabrics and hats became difficult.

THE BIGGER THE BETTER

In the 1910s, women wore their long hair in a bun or a chignon. Wearing your hair down was simply not done, unless you were a child. In true Edwardian spirit, the hair would be elegantly rolled up with lots of volume. Curling irons were heated by leaving them on the stove. To ensure the iron wasn't so hot it burned the hair off, women would hold a small piece of paper to the iron to test it. Clever—and frighteningly hazardous.

Once the updo was set, tiny wisps of hair were curled to showcase class and style. The pompous hairstyles stayed in place with U-shaped bobby pins and a tried-and-true technique—working with unwashed hair. This old hair-style trick still works well today.

Women then crowned their voluminous hairstyles with hats.

The general rule was that the bigger, more lavish, and more extraordinary the hat, the higher the woman's status. The brims were enormous and decorated with extravagant creations, featuring feathers, plumes, and silk flowers.

Fashion was just as severe as the hair buns, and very, very feminine. The silhouette was shaped like a curvy S, and buttons adorned virtually every garment. Hems reached just above the ankle. Sleeves were long (at the very least ¾-length) and corsets—which would soon be forgone—squeezed tight while collars reached high. Those who could afford them wore lace collars. A few years into the 1910s, collars became unbuttoned and less chaste, leaving room for new influences. Empire cuts, draped décolletages in delicate materials, bold patterns, and something as groundbreaking as color set the new fashion agenda. Inspiration came from East Asia. This elegant fashion spread like wildfire through the new ways of consumption. Department stores were a novelty. There, hats and scarves joined the company of something very new and bold: glass counters displaying cosmetics. Makeup itself was nothing new, but to sell it this openly—without the secretiveness that marked previous decades—was completely revolutionary. The prevalent all-natural beauty ideal forced women to apply makeup with great discretion. Both powder and blush were widely used, but in moderation. And in secret.

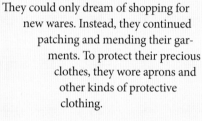

THE LAST DAYS OF CORSETS

At this time, the king of fashion, Paul Poiret, made his grand entrance. He made no secret of the fact that he was heavily influenced by East Asia and the Russian ballet company Les Ballets Russes. Slowly but surely, he liberated women from their corsets by introducing a tight skirt that became wildly popular. Paul Poiret is considered the first modern fashion designer. And though undergarments continued to be reminiscent of a suit of armor, Paul Poiret was among the first to bring his "liberating fashion" to the grand department stores.

For members of the working class, department stores were completely out of the question. They could only dream of shopping for new wares. Instead, they continued patching and mending their garments. To protect their precious clothes, they wore aprons and other kinds of protective clothing.

TRENDS IN TRANSITION

1910s fashion was narrow, tight, and uncomfortable. In fact, it was about as narrow as woman's role in society. But it didn't stay that way for much longer.

Women broke new ground as suffragettes, upsetting the system at hand. Until the 1910s, men had acted as women's guardians (this held true for a few more years), but at that point, women began to rebel. Fashion was gender-segregated and few dared to step (court shoe–clad) across gender boundaries.

Enter the groundbreaking Coco Chanel. Inspired by menswear, she presented a whole new look. Striped fishermen's shirts for women and—lo and behold—trousers. Her androgynous style would mean a lot in the decades thereafter and is still influential to this day.

THE 1920s

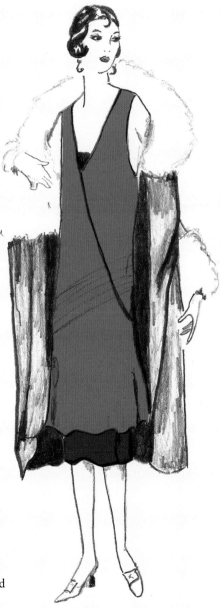

T he decadent and dramatic 1920s started off in an optimistic, future-embracing spirit. World War I was finally over and no one liked to dwell on the difficult years. It was the beginning of a new era.

To many people's chagrin, young women cut off their billowing long hair at the barber (hair salons for women were still not available). Daring short and feathered hairstyles paired with straight, calf-length dresses and swinging Charleston dancing became synonymous with a new and controversial female ideal. This is where our hairstyle history picks up.

Hair color to cover gray hair was introduced on the market, and the first attempts to bleach hair were carried out with less-than-perfect results.

The very short bob cut was born (the first real styled hairdo) and eyes were emphasized in sinful black, while thin, sharp lines marked the eyebrows and the mouth was painted small and deep red. This new ideal, rich in paint and contrasts, sprang from film. Sharp lines were created to make sure that facial features stood out on the silver screen, essential in this age of silent movies, when body language was used instead of speech.

Without a doubt, the cinema was the chief source of inspiration when it came to beauty, and remained so for the following decades.

The ideal was pale and androgynous, with a thin but important veneer of feminine decadence.

DARING FASHION

Finger Waves (page 50) and Faux Finger Waves (page 53) were styled when the short cuts were still soaking wet. As the name suggests, fingers (or a tail comb) were used to create this look. The short hairstyles were matched with straight dresses. The absence of a marked waistline was a novelty in the fashion history. Until this point, waists had either been corseted or, in the case of the empire cut, marked so high as to lead the gaze to the bust. In the 1920s, the focus on defined curves disappeared.

Corsets were abandoned. Instead, women bandaged their busts in order to create a seriously straight silhouette. The new titillating fashion brought attention to the skin: deep V-necks and dresses that fell just below the knee so that Charleston legs could move freely. Many emerging fashion designers found their inspiration in the world of sport. Jean Patou invented the knitted swimsuit and designed tennis clothes for women. Women, who had until then been expected to simply stand around and look beautiful, would finally have their own comfortable leisurewear.

Coco Chanel was an early proponent of this looser, more relaxed fashion. According to Mademoiselle Chanel, women should wear clothes that are so comfortable they shouldn't even have to think about what they're wearing. The startling designer stated that women had more important things on their minds, like laughing, eating (without fainting), and attaining the right to vote. Thus, clothing should be loose-fitting and free. All of this was wildly controversial. But the era's most famous and fashionable ladies stayed true to this spirit: Josephine Baker with her banana skirt, Clara Bow with her flirty appeal, and Marlene Dietrich in her sharp menswear.

FRONTLINE FLAPPERS
Over the dresses, loose coats (provokingly reminiscent of negligees) were worn, often adorned with fur details. It was all very decadent and glamorous—and utterly groundbreaking. Furthermore, many of the garments were sleeveless. Never before had women shown so much skin. The new fashion was simultaneously improper and refreshingly modern.

The flapper was born. These insolent, tomboyish women with short hair were both seen and heard. They smoked, drank absinthe, danced the Charleston, and demanded the right to vote. Pronto!

The color black became associated with fashion, rather than with grief. It was often paired with sharp hues of gold and silver. A new era had arrived.

Hair accessories were all the rage. Feathers, stones, and sequins adorned the chic hairstyles together with a thin ribbon delicately crowning the head. It was placed straight across the hairstyle—like a sweatband—with a carefully curved strand seemingly glued to the cheek. It was all very glamorous. For everyday life, women wore turbans, shawls, or cloche hats pulled down over the head, with a small but important strand of hair alluding to what was beneath the hat. It was during this time that the perm made its first appearance. It was not very successful, since it so often greatly damaged the hair. Metal curlers were used for these early perms, which in retrospect may seem quite an uncomfortable option.

But the best way to achieve the right 1920s look was by simply not washing one's hair. To get a fantastically glossy finish, hair grease and tonics were used. Hair pomade and sugar water were also common "products." For this look, hold was secondary. Instead, it was all about gloss, gloss, and more gloss. As more focus was placed on the hair, the world's first shampoo was launched. Until this point, ordinary soap had to do.

It was also during the Roaring '20s that the world saw the first electric curling iron. However, it was intended merely to give the hair waves, not to curl it.

THE 1930s

The merry laughter from the gay '20s faded into the less cheery 1930s, an era characterized by catastrophes veiled by unattainable glamour. The Wall Street crash of 1929 had a severe effect on the entire decade that followed. Recession was as deep as unemployment was high, and people escaped the hardships of everyday life by daydreaming about the infinitely glamorous world of Hollywood. They went to the movies.

The movie stars owned the world, and Jean Harlow was the queen of them all. She made way for a new trend when she starred in the movie *Platinum Blonde*. Bleached hair, preferably chin-length, was considered the ultimate in irresistible seduction. Bleaching one's hair with the new and trendy bleaching powder became a must.

With her long, cool curls, Veronica Lake swept onto the silver screen, leaving an iconic and everlasting imprint on the map of hairstyle fashions.

Women let their short, strict bob cuts from the 1920s grow out into long or semi-long hairstyles with billowing waves. Straight hair was suddenly considered improper. It was thought that hair should be curly or wavy, a trend that permeated hairstyle history until the 1960s.

COOL AND SENSUAL
Traditionally female shapes came back into fashion—the waist became marked again and skirts got longer. The fashion was alternately restrained, sensual, and cool. Dresses were cut deep in the back and fashioned out of delicate materials that revealed the contours of the body in a daringly modern way. For everyday life, coarser materials were used—but always with the female shapes in focus. Peplums graced coats and jackets to accentuate the female shape.

Greta Garbo dazzled in a suit with a long, flared skirt. She looked out from under her slouch hat with her legendary mysterious gaze. Hats were very popular during this period. They came in many inventive shapes, inspired by modern art. The rebellious Elsa Schiaparelli was a fashion pioneer. She created surreal hats and clothes. One of her most famous creations was a hat shaped like a shoe. She found her inspiration in the work of contemporary artists like Salvador Dalí.

13

The hat became the must-have accessory. During this time, there were more hat makers than coffee shops in Paris, the capital of fashion.

BIAS CUT: A 1930s CLASSIC

Alongside the functional suits, a new trend started to appear in the 1930s—long trousers. It was a whole new groundbreaking fashion rooted in the world of sport. The bias cut also became almost synonymous with '30s fashion. This diagonal cut, seen primarily in dresses, accentuated female shapes. Such dresses were made from fancy materials such as silk, and the bias cut fell beautifully. The silhouette was long and lean with sensual shapes.

The thin brows of the 1920s lived on for a decade while the rest of the makeup became more modest. The pale ideal, proving that one was not out working hard in the fields, was replaced by a "healthy" slightly tanned look. In summertime, women bared skin when outdoors—a behavior considered unacceptable until then. In this sun-kissed era, the first sunscreen was launched, leaving a delicately scented trace of roses and jasmine.

INVENTIVE TIMES

As the Depression deepened, fashion became more inventive. Women saved, mended, dyed, and refashioned their garments.

When it came to matters of hair, things truly started changing. The primitive and positively lethal hair-styling tools of the past century were tucked away. Instead, women began to style their hair using Pin Curls (page 34), an effective way of curling the hair when you're out of money, since all you need are bobby pins. Another budget-savvy way of curling your hair was to make rag curls. With this method, you simply rolled your hair on what you happened to have at home, such as rags. Despite the meager means, it was during the 1930s that hair products really started to appear on the market. Toward the end of the 1930s, modern chemicals came into use for curling hair in so-called perms.

As Billie Holiday sang "Summertime" with her pin-curled hair, people started dreaming of a better tomorrow. Of a future where they weren't struggling to get by in worn-out socks.

THE 1940s

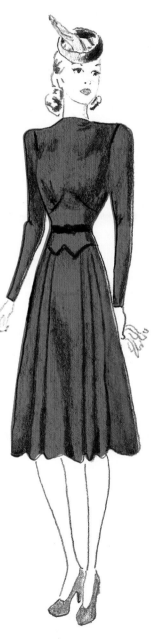

With bombs and grenades falling, World War II had the world in a tight grip.

As men reported for military duty, women were encouraged to seek employment. They left their unpaid labor by the stove to go make their own money in factories and offices.

They clitter-clattered into the work market and made a noticeable impact on society in many ways. For instance, fashion found inspiration in uniforms, and it turned toward the more practical and often masculine. No wonder, since many of the new clothes for women were made out of fabric from men's clothing.

The cool, sensual shapes of the 1930s were flattened into a square silhouette where broad power shoulders and slim, slightly flared skirts made up the uniform of the era. Military details such as epaulettes and brass buttons were in focus, together with the sturdy work wear of the factory floors. Rough and durable fabrics like wool were trademarks of the '40s. Fabric was used with utmost care and economy, resulting in an increasingly figure-hugging fashion. In these rationing times, skirts got just a little bit shorter and dresses were cut with nary a millimeter to spare—anything to get the most out of the expensive materials.

STOCKINGS AS STATUS SYMBOLS

Long socks were traded for more rationing-friendly shorter ones. A small number of privileged ladies wore nylon stockings with a fancy seam in the back. Should there ever be a run in the stocking, it was promptly mended with care and special tools. Ladies who were not fortunate enough to have seamed nylons simply drew a line on the backs of their legs. And in a flash, they created an illusion of owning the desired goods and kept their status intact.

Since it was considered indecent to walk around with bare legs, new demands for creativity were born. So-called leg art—color to be painted straight onto bare legs—was a new phenomenon invented during these tough, rationing times.

Besides legs, women also painted their lips. Strong eyebrows and red lipstick characterized the decade. Lipstick became a symbol of power and strength (see page 107) and was one of the few items considered an acceptable purchase given the hard-pressed economy.

HAIR: THE MOST AFFORDABLE ACCESSORY OF THE CENTURY

Never-ending creativity and resourcefulness were synonymous with times of crisis in general, and with World War II in particular. Times may have been tight, but ideas abounded. Recycling was a given, as there was no other alternative.

During these meager war years, it was considered shameful to waste any scarce items such as fabric, buttons, or thread. As both wardrobes and wallets gaped empty, attention was directed to what women did have—hair. You would have to look very hard to find a cheaper accessory! Spectacular hairstyles became the hottest accessories of the era. In order to create such hairdos, many women grew their hair a little longer, but not too long. Shoulder length was the ideal— the perfect length for creating the hairstyles of the day and just the right length to gather into a simple roll at the nape of your neck. Within some professions, hair was not even allowed to touch the collar. You can see some of these styles on pages 43, 45, and 68.

Hair buns or fillers were also used to create voluminous styles. These could be made from your own hair, simply gathered and rolled together. This very natural filler was then placed inside your hair for that extra boost.

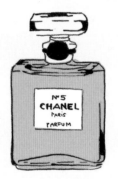

DARK AND CURLY

Hair ideally was curly. If you didn't have natural curls, you could achieve them with the help of pin curls or metal rollers. Curly hair made it easier to create the hairstyles of the time; straight hair would not be socially accepted for decades to come. During this period, the chemical perm gained in popularity, just as dyes and bleaches did. The blonde ideal that had characterized the 1930s was traded for a darker look. Now every woman and girl dreamed of looking like red-headed Lucille Ball or the beautiful and strong, trouser-wearing Katharine Hepburn.

HAIR AS HOBBY

In the gloomy days of World War II rationing, a new hobby began to emerge. Instead of knitting or crocheting from rationed, expensive products, women's creativity found a new outlet in a brand-new budget hobby: hairstyling. To turn a friend's hair into an artistic 'do was the 1940s version of today's DIY craze. At that point in time, two revolutionary products were introduced on the market: setting lotion and hair spray.

As the last sounds of bullets faded away, the "V for Victory" message made its proud entry into the world. The V-signs were seen everywhere. On pins and flyers . . . and in hairstyles such as the Victory Rolls (page 60). Hair was styled into rolls, shaping a proud V-shaped message to announce that the war was over.

THE NEW LOOK

In 1947, Christian Dior introduced his world-famous hourglass silhouette, "The New Look." It became the starting point for exactly what the term implies—a brand-new ideal. The days of uniform-inspired fashion were over. Masculine shapes were exchanged for rounder, more feminine ones. The skirts become wider, while waistlines were tightened.

Women headed back to their unpaid work by the stove, dressed in clothes that were far from practical. Women were no longer supposed to be employed or save the world. The new ambition—being drop-dead gorgeous— was clearly reflected in fashion.

THE 1950s

A brighter future was just around the corner. No one wanted to look back now that war and worry were over. It was all about looking ahead. The men returned to the factories, and women put their overalls and scarves away. With their hair perfectly set and their nails freshly painted, they were far away from the dust and grease of the factory floors.

The expectation for the 1950s woman was to be a representative housewife, moving around the house in close proximity to a refrigerator and vacuum cleaner. A well-managed home with a wife by the stove was proof of a man's success.

The rationing times with coupons and thin wallets now over, paychecks grew more generous and the standard of living increased for both men and their wives. Suitcases were packed with novelties such as the bikini, and vacations were inspired by catchy slogans like "To Paris and Such . . . KLM Royal Dutch."

The affluence of the times and the great hopes for the future were reflected in the world of fashion and beauty. There was an abundance of bright pastels, luxury, and feminine shapes. Christian Dior's "New Look" from 1947 dominated the fashion scene of the 1950s. To this day, it remains the style ideal we see when we look back on this decade.

THE CORSET COMEBACK

Femininity and the female form played a key role in the fashion of the era. It was not unusual to use 30 yards of fabric to make a wide skirt, or to use scraps of fabric for the itty-bitty waist. The waist was tightened with corsets and girdles to create the desirable "wasp waist."

The bust was pushed upward and sculpted into a sharp, perky shape with a bra. Dresses had built-in metal wiring to ensure ideal curves. In order to emphasize hips, petticoats were starched with sugar or potato flour to bump up the full skirts. The very wide shoulders, so fashionable in the 1940s, gave way to the more disarming, sloping, and narrow-shouldered silhouette.

To further enhance this look, women wore boat-necked designs and coats with three-quarter dropdown sleeves. Fashion-savvy ladies added gloves and a purse to complete the ensemble.

The female ideal was candidly innocent yet brassy, like Marilyn Monroe or Diana Dors. They peeked out from under their bangs with arched brows, generously winged eyeliner, and eyelashes painted with roll-on mascara. And pouting red lips to match.

After the war, a number of new beauty products were introduced: liquid eyeliner, compact powder, pastel eye shadows, and pancake makeup—all beautifully packaged and stored in the new must-have for women: the beauty box.

CANDY-COLORED CURLERS

Hair was cut and curled or gathered into a graceful ponytail (see page 88). The complicated hairstyles that characterized the previous decade got combed out into polished, set 'dos.

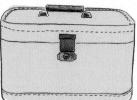

Curls were still an important status symbol, but there were more ways of achieving them than simply using pin curls. Plastic curlers hit the market—a small revolution! If you looked closely, you could catch a glimpse of pastel curlers beneath the hairnets. They were worn Monday through Friday, then let out in time for the weekend, revealing a fresh set of beautiful curls. A quick spray to fix the 'do and you're set for afternoon tea.

In the new, more affluent society, many people could afford a trip to the hair salon. Naturally, this showed. Going to the hairstylist was common and necessary to keep the new short styles looking sleek.

For festive occasions, the hair was styled in upswept 'dos like the Pile of Curls (page 56) or in a Poodle with Sweep-Up (page 64). Bangs played an increasingly important part when it came to hairstyles. They came in many shapes. Audrey Hepburn and Brigitte Bardot both made bangs an essential part of their signature looks, each with her own individual take on the fringe.

In 1951, a new kind of hair color was introduced to the market. For the first time, this dye didn't require the hair to be bleached prior to coloring. Furthermore, the first tint became readily available. These tubes of color paved the way for our current colors and tints. During this time, Technicolor revolutionized the movie world with its vibrant colors. In its wake, a new hair color trend was born. Mild or meek colors had no place in this colorful era. Fiery red, platinum blonde, and raven black were eye-catching colors setting the trend.

Silver shampoo was also a product of this era, as was the light plastic hair dryer (until this point, dryers had been heavy and ungainly metal appliances). The hat, which had been a must, got a makeover. The pillbox hat (page 98) or a birdcage hat (page 101), elegantly balanced on the back of the head, was a perfect match for short, curled hair.

REBELS AND ROCK 'N' ROLL

A new generation of youngsters grew up in the midst of rosebushes, homemade pies, and Tupperware. They chewed gum, listened to rock 'n' roll, and were rebels in denim and leather jackets. Up to this point, young people had dressed in junior versions of men's and women's fashion. It was not till the 1960s that a distinctive youth fashion began to emerge, breaking free from a world of shiny kitchen counters and set hair. With the new youth movement, numerous style directions were born. Among them were beatniks: young rebels who wanted to change the world. They dressed in black turtlenecks, slacks, and berets (see page 89) and looked just like Audrey Hepburn in *Funny Face*. Sinfully black hair in a ponytail and bangs with an attitude became the signature look and hairstyle of the young rebel.

THE 1960s

A new rebellious youth culture emerged out of the prim and proper 1950s. A generation that had grown up in suburban row-house communities with shiny, candy-colored cars looked over and beyond the white picket fences, facing a postwar era that was far from the delightful reality everyone had hoped for.

In the wake of the war, a frosty climate put a shuddering film over everyday life. Fears waited just around the corner. The world's superpowers flexed their muscles like rivals in a sweaty bodybuilder competition. They began to compare their respective strengths and armed themselves for an uncertain future while polishing the iron curtain.

Meanwhile, fighting grew increasingly intense in Vietnam. After the TV became a staple in every household during the '50s, images from a war-ravaged Asia spread across the world in an unprecedented way. The Vietnam War was the first televised war, and reactions were instantaneous. The moving images awakened sympathy, and young people refused to watch contently from their shiny diner seats. Instead, they hit the streets and squares to express their discontent. Together they were strong—and they were many. Protests became a new way of expression for an upset generation.

SMALL, MEDIUM, LARGE:
A MORE LIBERAL TAKE ON FASHION

The 1960s were a decade when everything seemed possible—including traveling to the moon—so why not create a whole new world? The youth rebellion was in motion.

Set to the tunes of pop and rock 'n' roll, the world should've been democratic and freed from violence and war. But the world couldn't be saved in crisp, gauzy taffeta with a corset and set curls. In the name of freedom, a new fashion was born. Expensive pieces, tailored to fit the unique and personal measurements of an individual, gave way to democratic, mass-produced garments. People started to be divided into generic sizes: small, medium, and large.

Beatlemania enveloped the world, and suddenly all eyes were on Carnaby Street and the fashion mecca of the 1960s: swinging London. Streets become the new catwalk and music was the outer seam of youth fashion. Shapes got straighter and shorter. In 1964, Mary Quant designed the first miniskirt, and though short from the beginning, it just kept getting shorter. In the end, it was just 12 inches/30.5 centimeters "long"—roughly the length of a regular school ruler. Minis were in, as were Peter Pan collars and graphic prints. Pop art reigned supreme, with Andy Warhol and the Factory as its king. By Warhol's side stood muse Edie Sedgwick with her graphically made-up eyes and platinum blonde hair.

YOUR SUBCULTURE DECIDES YOUR 'DO

Never before had fashion been so expressive, influential, or multifaceted. Suddenly, there were infinite styles to choose from when it came to fashion and hair, depending on which subculture you identified with and which hairstylist you saw. During the 1960s, an ever-growing number of hairdressers graduated from beauty schools, and the hairdressing chairs lined up accordingly. British-born Vidal Sassoon created groundbreaking fashion hairstyles designed to match Mary Quant's miniskirted lines, while Frenchman Alexandre Raimon created elegant updos, such as Elizabeth Taylor's hairstyle in the movie *Cleopatra*. One 1960s novelty was the new wash-and-wear 'do, cut to flatter the shape of the face. Another novelty was the teased beehive, which grew bigger and bigger.

CURLY GOES STRAIGHT

Straight hair enjoyed a comeback. For decades, curly hair had been highly prized, but in the '60s pin curls, rag curls, perms, and curling irons were tucked away. They were considered a thing of the past, associated with the older generations. Hair should be straight and shiny, though a natural wave might pass. In order to make the hair stay in place, novelties such as hair gel were introduced.

The sophisticated curls of the 1950s were combed out into a long and shiny Catherine Deneuve 'do, a Jackie Flip (page 86), tousled Brigitte Bardot hair, a voluminous Beehive (page 84), or a geometric, sharp bob. And last—but not least—the pixie cut, the signature look of the great icon of the decade: Twiggy. With the exception of Mademoiselle Bardot, the round, feminine shapes were cast away and just about everyone wanted to look like the reed-thin model Twiggy.

A childish look was all the rage. Women wore knee-high socks and baby doll dresses that suited flat, straight bodies.

The makeup was all about the eyes. The right look was achieved with eyeliner, emphasized crease lines, and mink eyelashes (see page 106). The focus on the eyes was balanced by a light touch of blush and bare lips.

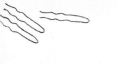

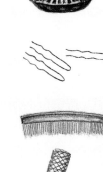
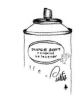

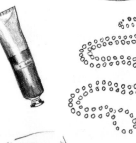
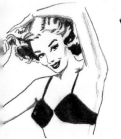
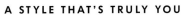
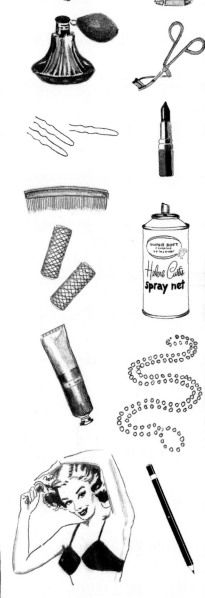

A STYLE THAT'S TRULY YOU

*Today, we have the privilege of dressing
how we choose. We can wear a 1960s
frock one day and a 1930s outfit the
next. We live in an age when fashion is
wonderfully accepting. We can pick up
on the fancies of yesteryear to create
something entirely our own. Whether
you decide to strictly stick to the style
of just one era or mix and match as you
go, playing around with the fashion
of bygone eras often leads to a
style that's uniquely you.*

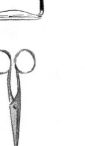

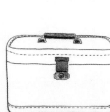
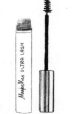

Tools and Tips

OF THE TRADE

DON'T WASTE HOURS SITTING UNDER THE DRYER HOOD! CREATE YOUR OWN VINTAGE HAIRSTYLE IN A FLASH WITH SMART TOOLS AND HANDS-ON ADVICE!

Thanks to new tools and products, we now have the luxury of creating beautiful old-school 'dos in just a third of the time it used to take back in the day. Naturally, some of you will still choose pin curls and rollers, but there are speedier ways to get the look right.

Both tools and hair products have been modified over the years, enabling women to build careers, realize dreams, and spend time on a sea of hobbies while simultaneously looking great. This is a welcome development in a world where each and every moment is captured for posterity.

Instead of heating your curling iron on the stove (and repeating the process over and over as the iron cools off), you can simply plug your electric iron into an outlet. Five to ten minutes, a few spritzes of hair spray, and you're done. You don't even have to sleep on hard, uncomfortable curlers.

In addition, hair doesn't need to suffer the kind of damage that styling used to cause. These days, there are products like heat protectants, hair oil, and hair masks to keep your hair healthy as you create beautiful vintage-inspired creations.

Even hygiene has advanced. In our wonderfully scented, shampooed world of hair care, hair is washed more often (thankfully), though we could often benefit from waiting another day or two. When it comes to creating great hairstyles, the ideal hair is slightly unwashed.

Women used to leave their hair unwashed for weeks on end. Instead, they used dry shampoos made from baking powder or corn flour. Today, dry shampoo has enjoyed a glorious comeback and is readily available in pretty cans and stylish bottles. The main principle remains: Dry shampoo should dust off the hair, removing the unwashed finish. This is a tactic that has been popular for hundreds of years and still works. These days, dry shampoo is used both to freshen hair and to increase volume and hold, especially when it comes to updos.

To make these beautiful vintage hairstyles, we've translated old techniques into more modern versions. Through new methods, products, and innovations, we'll teach you how to go about creating the most wonderful styles.

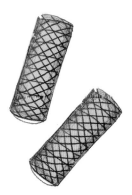

OUR BEST TRICKS AND TIPS

• Stand in front of a mirror and lift your hair up around your head. Move it around and play with the hair to see what styles, lengths, and shapes best suit your face.

• Each person's hair is different and naturally falls in its own way. Try to work with your hair's natural style to save both time and effort.

• When going to bed, put a hairnet over your 'do. The next day, your hair will be a little bit messy but still just as stylish. Recycling!

• Wiggle bobby pins right under the hair surface to make them less visible.

• Try to spray hair spray on the "back" of tiny flyaway hairs, then gently pat them in place. Spraying them from above only makes them more prone to rebel.

• Busy morning? Curl your hair the night before and roll it up in Pin Curls (page 34). The next day, all you have to do is let down your curls, brush a little, and voilà! Your hair looks freshly done.

23

HAIRSTYLES AND
FACE SHAPES

Which hairstyle is the ideal fit for your face shape?
Find your perfect match.

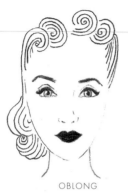

OBLONG

+ style with volume from
  cheekbone
− avoid upward volume

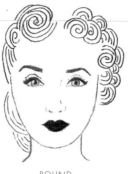

ROUND

+ try longer styles
− avoid round, puffy styles

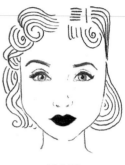

SQUARE

+ try soft shapes
− avoid hard shapes

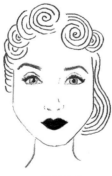

TRIANGLE

+ style with upward volume
− avoid volume around
  cheekbones

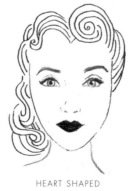

HEART SHAPED

+ style with loops that
  balance the heart shape
− avoid upward volume

OVAL

+ most styles work
− avoid volume upward
  and downward

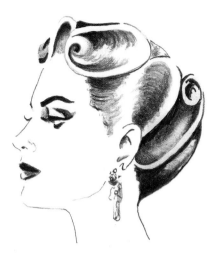

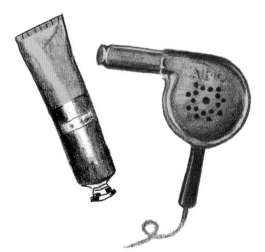

ON YOUR DRESSING TABLE

Prepare your new vintage self by equipping your dressing table with a few select hairstyle necessities, such as brushes, combs, clips, and pins. Read on for our hairstyle must-haves.

ESSENTIAL TOOLS

What you need for the perfect hairstyle

HEAT PROTECTANTS

As the name implies, heat protectants shield your hair from the heat of curling irons and flat irons, which cause terrible damage to the hair. Heat protection is built into many mousses, setting lotions, gels, and creams, but there are also no-hold heat protectants. These often come in spray cans.

HOT ROLLERS

Use hot rollers to create beautiful volume or to prep the hair prior to styling an updo.

CURLING IRON OR FLAT IRON

These tools can fix your curls in a hurry, but the result doesn't hold as long as Pin Curls (page 34) or Rollers (page 36).

FOAM ROLLERS

If you're after smaller, firmer curls, go for foam rollers or bendy rollers. Foam rollers are relatively comfortable to wear when you sleep, if you'd like to try overnight curling.

WAVE CLIPS

Use these clips when you're making Finger Waves (page 49). Instead of relying solely on your fingers (as the name implies), these clips help shape the waves.

SETTING LOTION/SETTING GEL

Use setting lotion to make your curls last longer. Setting lotion also makes flyaways more manageable.

POMADE/GLOSSING CREAM

Add shine and shape to your curls with products like pomade, glossing cream, or glossing spray. It helps add that little extra spark to your 'do. Apply these products before you set the style with hair spray.

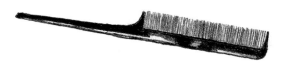

TAIL COMB

A tail comb is a must on the dressing table. It's useful for many tasks, such as sectioning and teasing, and is a great tool when setting your hair.

NATURAL BRISTLE BRUSH

A brush with soft, dense natural bristles is a great help when brushing out your curls. This brush shapes and smooths the hair and helps create cool and sensual 1930s curls.

STYLING BRUSH

This rounded brush with close-set plastic bristles often comes with a rubber base and a plastic handle. It's useful for brushing out your hair after setting as well as for making stylish updos and blowouts.

BOBBY PINS

Bobby pins have many uses when it comes to vintage hairstyling. Perfect for pin curls and all kinds of updos.

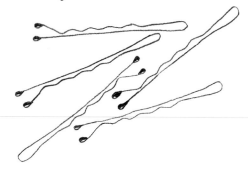

HAIR CLIPS

Hair clips are clips that hold the hair in place. They are usually plastic or metal and can be used while you style your hair or to create hairstyles.

HAIR COMBS

Hair combs, which are used to hold the hair in place, are often plastic or metal, and might be plain or embellished.

U-PINS

U-pins are a must for buns and chignons. They spread out the hair and keep it in place. They are also great when you want to secure single sections of hair.

FILLERS/HAIR BUNS/HAIR PADS

Filler products come in handy when you want to increase volume as you make a roll or a French Twist (page 76). They are also great when making Faux Bettie Bangs (page 42).

THIN HAIRNETS

Hairnets are perfect for those humid days when you fear your curls are not holding. A fine-mesh hairnet is barely visible and works great if you want to create a shorter style for a day. Hairnets are also ideal when making longer-hair updos.

SETTING NET

Use a setting net when drying your curls. It lets air come through while keeping your pin curls or rollers in place during the night.

HAIR SPRAY

Set styles and 'dos with hair spray, the most essential of all hair products. Use hair spray at the very end of your hairstyling process to control small hairs and to achieve a perfect finish.

DRY SHAMPOO

Dry shampoo has been around for decades. These days, it's a favorite both in salons and on dressing tables. The powder increases volume while simultaneously de-shining unwashed hair. Furthermore, dry shampoo gives better hold, which is ideal when it comes to creating updos.

ACCESSORIES

Flowers, scarves, jewelry, feathers, combs, and ribbons can all be put to use to create truly unique and creative styles. See pages 98–101 for handy tips on how to make your own pretty yet simple accessories.

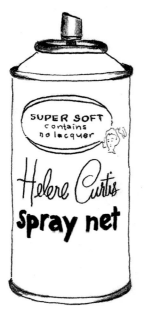

SUPER SOFT
contains
no lacquer

Helene Curtis
spray net

Plan Your Hair Days

14 MONDAY
Day 1. Just washed hair. Let hair down with a fresh set of curls. At night, hairnet.

15 TUESDAY
Day 2. Dry shampoo and re-brush, or make a partial updo.

16 WEDNESDAY
Day 3. Time for an updo!

THURSDAY 17
Day 4. Scarf!

FRIDAY 18

19 SATURDAY

SUNDAY 20

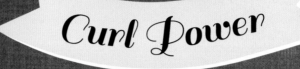

Curl Power

TECHNIQUES FOR CURLY LOCKS

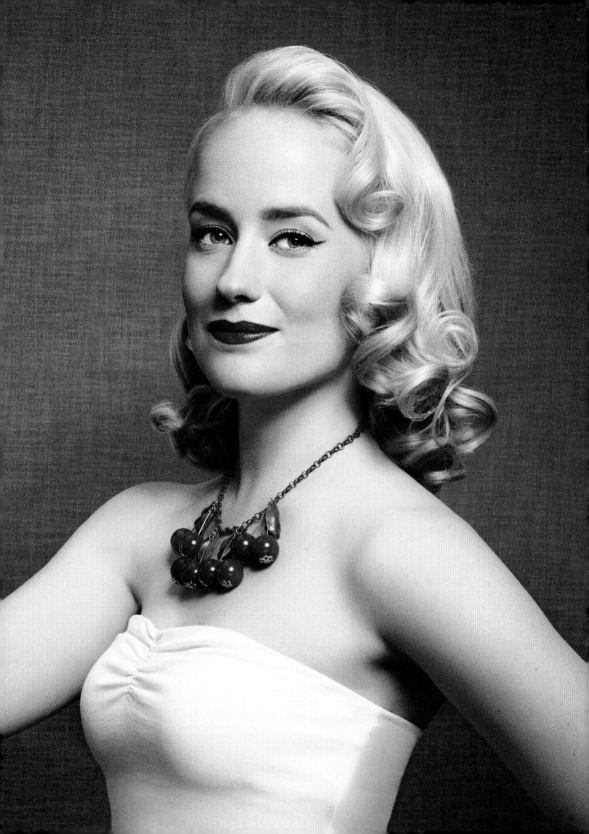

CURLS FOR ALL TIMES

FIVE-MINUTE CURLS OR PIN CURLS THAT DO
THE WORK WHILE YOU SLEEP? FIND YOUR
FAVORITE AND LEARN HOW TO MAKE
YOUR CURLS LAST LONGER.

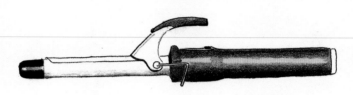

Elegant waves, crimped 1930s locks, a round and voluminous 1950s bounce, or a 1960s flip—curly hair is the foundation of all vintage hair; a must, at least historically speaking.

Back in the day, women would go to the hair salon to get their hair set. Straight hair was considered unattractive, untidy, and bordering on unfeminine, which was practically considered a derogatory remark at the beginning of the twentieth century. As soon as femininity seemed to be at risk, the public responded with an outcry. It didn't matter if traditional womanhood was presumably under attack because of trousers, tops that didn't accentuate the bust, or cropped hair. Popular fury did not discriminate.

But despite all those pants-wearing, straight-haired threats, women have survived well into the twenty-first century. These days, we enjoy being so liberated that we can wear our hair straight or curly. Should we choose curls, we can do it easily and for our own reasons.

For example, we can curl our hair because it's beautiful or because it's a great start for any updo. To help us, we have innovations like curling irons or flat irons with their promise of beautiful curls

just a cord's length away. However, old-school methods, paired with new products, are becoming increasingly popular.

In the past, curls were created with perms, different kinds of rollers (see page 36), Pin Curls (page 34), or curling irons. The first curling irons were heated over open fire or simply put on top of the stove. Many a woman had her hair ruined because the heat control was so limited. In 1959, the first electric curling iron was launched, a truly revolutionary invention. There have also been numerous kinds of rollers. At first, rollers were heavy and made from metal. Toward mid-century, they were replaced by plastic rollers and foam rollers. Plastic curlers reigned supreme.

During the 1940s and 1950s, hair was curled with pin curls—an inexpensive, accessible, and effective way to achieve curls that first appeared in the 1930s. Women rolled up their wet hair into loops and then left it to dry overnight or under a hairnet while they took care of everyday chores. One of these pin curl–loving females was Marilyn Monroe. It's true—the blonde bombshell created her world-famous look with the help of pin curls.

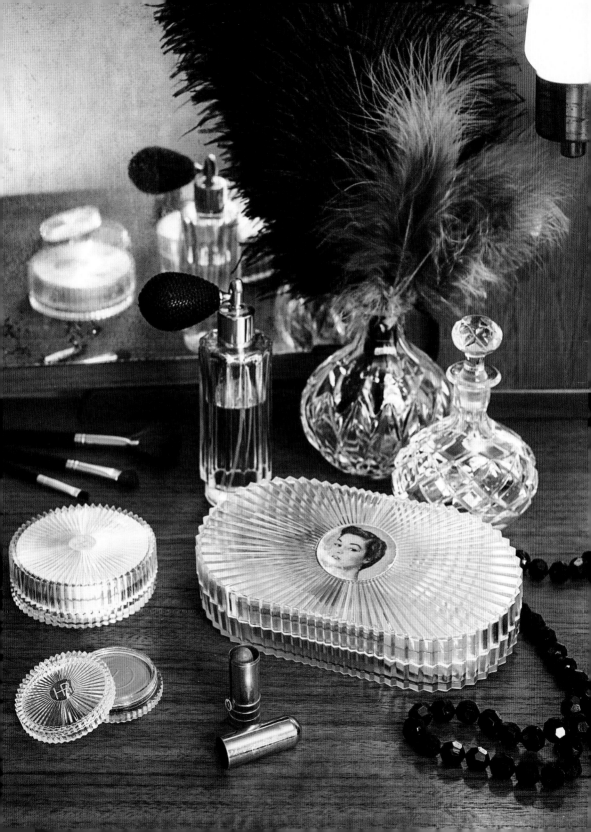

FLAT IRON

Pull hair through an angled flat iron and create curly hair in just a minute!

STYLING BRUSH
HEAT PROTECTANT
FLAT IRON
BOBBY PINS

1. Before you get started, make sure the hair is completely dry. Brush through the hair thoroughly to make the iron glide more easily. Prepping the hair with a heat protectant is a great idea, especially if the protectant provides some kind of hold.

2. Gather a section of hair, not too thick, so the heat from the flat iron can reach all the way through. If you're going for a look reminiscent of the 1920s through 1950s, always curl inward so that the ends of the hair are turned toward your face. If you curl outward, you'll end up with a style that is more inspired by the '60s or '70s. Try to decide what look you're after before you get started. Once you start curling, changing direction can be a bit tricky.

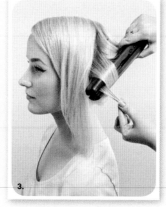

3.

3. Gently bring the flat iron tongs together over the hair. Start 1 in/2.5 cm up from the scalp to make sure you don't accidentally burn yourself. This little distance will also make it easier to angle the iron. Turn the iron inward for a whole turn (360 degrees). Shift your hold after half a turn to make it easier to handle the iron. You know you've made a complete turn once the hair ends point downward again. Then slowly pull the flat iron straight down and all the way out to the very ends of the hair section, and voilà, a curl is born.

4. Roll the curl up into a Pin Curl (page 34) and set with bobby pins or hair clips or let it cool off on its own. Don't pull on the hair while it's hot or it will lose its bounce. For maximum spring and hold, let the curl cool as a pin curl.

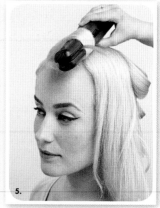

5.

5. To increase bangs volume, curl by pulling the section of hair straight up. Start 1 in/2.5 cm from the scalp, rotate a full turn (360 degrees), and then pull straight out.

Note: You create more or less volume depending on what angle you hold the iron and in which direction you pull. For maximum volume, pull straight up. If you pull straight out, you'll achieve medium volume, while pulling straight down will result in just a little volume.

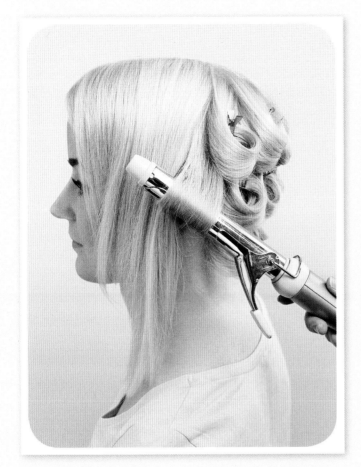

CURLING IRON

As easy as roll up and hold! This tool has been around for thousands of years and continues to be a curl favorite to this day. Thankfully, the adjustable heat settings of modern irons mean we've come a long way from the burned hair of bygone irons.

You'll need

STYLING BRUSH
HEAT PROTECTANT
CURLING IRON
HAIR CLIPS

1. Be sure the hair is completely dry before you get started. Brush through the hair thoroughly to make the iron glide more easily. As with a flat iron, prepping the hair with a heat protectant is always a plus, particularly it it provides some kind of hold.

2. Take a small section of hair, about 1 in/2.5 cm. The smaller the section, the firmer the curl. Place the section at the outer end of the iron and let the tongs take hold of the hair. Then roll the iron almost all the way in to the scalp. Hold.

3. Touch the hair and assess. Has the heat permeated through the entire section to the outermost layer? If so, release the tongs. Fasten as you would a pin curl (page 34) and let cool or simply let it loose.

As with a flat iron, the angle of your iron determines the volume of the curl. If you roll the section straight up you'll end up with lots of volume. Roll horizontally to create medium volume, and roll vertically for less volume.

PIN CURLS

All you need to make pin curls are bobby pins. And time. Pin curls result in extremely durable curls and have been a favorite since the 1930s.

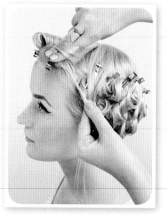

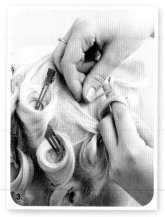

You'll need

SETTING LOTION, GEL, OR MOUSSE
TAIL COMB
HAIR CLIPS OR BOBBY PINS
HAIRNET OR SCARF
STYLING BRUSH

1. Make sure hair is damp before you get started. Apply setting lotion, gel, or mousse to wet hair. It will increase curl hold.

2. Gather a section of hair from around the temples with a tail comb. Have fine hair? Gather a somewhat larger section of hair. Have thick hair? Go for smaller sections.

3. Take hold of the hair and place one, two, or three fingers (one finger for small curls, two for medium curls, and three for large curls) 1 in/2.5 cm from the scalp, then wind the hair up on your finger(s). Let your right hand act as a spool on your left side and vice versa.

Keep winding until you only have the very ends of the hair left. Gently remove your fingers.

Tips!

• *Want to keep your curls looking great for a second day? Do a few bigger pin curls in the evening on dry hair to maintain your curls. Or sleep with a hairnet on.*

• *Did one of your locks lose its curl? Make a pin curl and flatten it gently with the flat iron to help it bounce back into shape.*

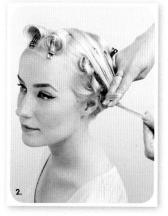

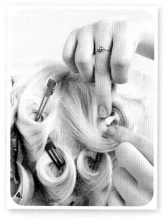

4. Roll the very last bit of hair in like a wheel, and then tip the pin curl toward the back so that the hair ends are placed against the head, between the scalp and the pin curl. Secure with a clip or a bobby pin straight across the pin curl.

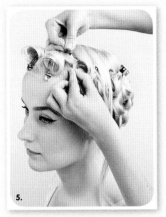

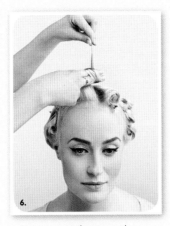

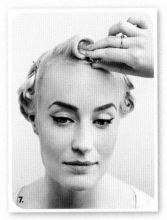

5. Work your way back from the side pin curls. Divide the remaining hair in one, two, or three rows depending on how much hair you have and how much volume you'd like to create.

The direction of the pin curls decreases in importance the further back you work. Alternate the rolling direction as you go.

6. To create voluminous bangs, make upright pin curls. Hold a section of hair straight up as you start rolling around your finger(s). Once you've rolled the entire section (including the ends), keep the pin curl vertical, or upright.

7. Secure the curl with a hair clip or a bobby pin inside the loop instead of across the curl. Cover the pin curls with a hairnet or a thin scarf to protect your curls while they dry—during the day or while you sleep.

When it's time to let the curls out, make sure they are entirely dry, otherwise they may not fully set. Remove the pins from the curls. See page 37 for brushing out and finishing.

Want Them Wavy?

If you're yearning for wavy bangs, pin the curls flat against your head instead of upright. Alternate the direction of the curl in each row. Brush out as described on page 37 and in the section on Large Billowing Waves (page 52).

ROLLERS

Rollers or curlers are trusted classics when it comes to curls. Roll up, wait—all done!

SETTING LOTION, GEL, OR MOUSSE
TAIL COMB
ROLLERS
HAIRNET OR SCARF
STYLING BRUSH

1. Begin with damp hair— preferably prepped with setting lotion, gel, or mousse— to ensure your curls achieve great hold and last longer.

2. Gather a section of hair with a tail comb. Pull the tail comb tip horizontally across the scalp to gather a section of hair roughly as wide as the roller. Depending on how much volume you'd like to create, choose in which direction you roll. Roll straight up for maximum volume, straight out for medium volume, and straight down for less volume.

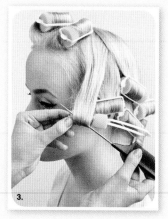

3.

3. Start rolling from the hair tips, stopping only to tuck little hairs into the roll with the tail comb. Roll all the way up.

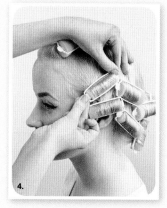

4.

4. If using foam rollers, snap the frame shut. Foam rollers permit more variation than other rollers. For instance, you can choose to roll just halfway or all the way. Velvet rollers and curlers should always be rolled all the way, then secured in place with a plastic pin pushed through the curler in a slanted upward direction.

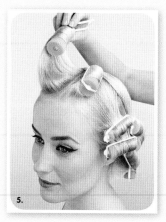

5.

5. The pictures show how to roll a typical 1940s style. Roll the hair straight up and down, that is to say not at an angle, with the exception of the bangs. To create a more 1950s-inspired look, roll curlers at the crown of the head as well, but straight up or straight out on the sides. The objective is to create maximum volume. Let hair dry overnight in a hairnet or during the day under a scarf. Once hair is completely dry, remove rollers and brush out according to the directions on the opposite page. Not quite dry? Use a hair dryer before brushing out.

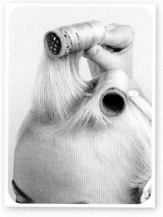

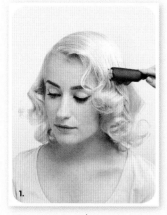

1.

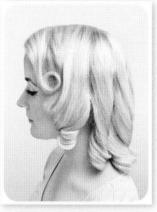

1. Remove any clips, pins, or rollers from hair. Brush straight down, using a natural bristle brush. Make sure the hair is brushed through completely—there should be no tangles or knots.

BRUSHING OUT

Turn ringlets into beautiful Veronica Lake–style vintage waves. All you need is a brush and a few tricks.

You'll need

NATURAL BRISTLE BRUSH
STYLING BRUSH
HAIR CREAM OR LIGHT WAX
TAIL COMB
HAIR SPRAY

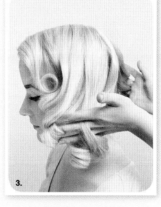

3.

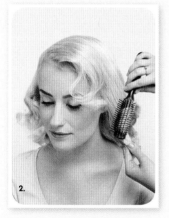

2.

2. Part the hair into several small sections, then brush each section with a styling brush. Brush each section several times. Always brush from the underside of the hair, angling the brush to achieve the desired curl shape. Brush ends inward to achieve 1940s- and 1950s-inspired 'dos and outward for a more 1960s look.

3. Keep brushing all the way around the head, then separate the curls with your fingers. If your hair tends to get frizzy, apply a small amount of hair cream or light wax to your fingers before you start. Use just a small dab; whichever product you're using shouldn't weigh down the hair. Shape curls in your preferred style. The more you separate the curls, the more volume you'll get.

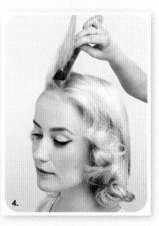

4.

4. Use a tail comb to tease the hair closest to the scalp in places where you'd like to create more volume. Brush tiny hairs into place. Once you're happy with your look, spray to set the style.

Protect Your Curls

Making sure curls stay bouncy and
beautiful all day is not always a walk
in the park. Rain and wind make it
even harder. Avoid limp curls
by remembering our
guidelines.

HANDY TIPS FOR LONGER-LASTING CURLS

PRODUCTS

In humid weather, use more setting lotion. Mousse and gel work great, too, as long as you increase the amount a bit.

Mist hair with hair spray. Try to do several thin coats instead of just one big dousing. Hair spray applied this way results in a great, weatherproof hold.

HAIRNET

Go for a fine, almost invisible net or a snood, which is also beautiful as an accessory. Want to make sure your hair looks dazzling in the evening? Wear a hairnet all day long. There are so many different hairnets on the market; choose between invisible (available in a number of natural colors) and bright and colorful varieties that do the job while doubling as a nice accessory.

HEADSCARF

Bring this forgotten accessory back on the scene—it's wonderfully protective of your curls. It's perfect when rain is spattering and your umbrella fails to help. Plus, a scarf is easy to bring with you, a portable hardworking hero that takes up very little space in a handbag. Wrap once around your head, then once around your neck.

THREE RAINY DAY FAVES

•

HAIR SPRAY
HAIRNET
SCARF

•

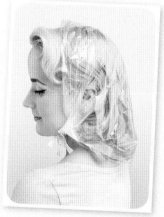

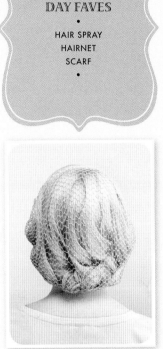

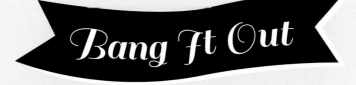

Bang It Out

GIVE YOUR BANGS A TOUCH OF VINTAGE GLAMOUR. DON'T HAVE ACTUAL BANGS? FAKE IT TILL YOU MAKE IT. HERE ARE SOME TIPS ON HOW TO VARY YOUR BANGS.

Bangs are a recurring trend. Historically speaking, very sharp bangs made their first appearance in the 1920s, when they were ideally straight, preferably matched with a bob cut, and slightly flattened by a cloche hat. In the 1930s, long bangs were combed in a daring side part. It was far from a fringed era. In the 1940s, sensual side parts gave way to pin-curl bangs. In the 1950s, pinup queen Bettie Page appeared on the scene with her round, polished bangs. Bettie's bangs became trendsetting along with the short, side-swept style worn by Audrey Hepburn.

But the true big bang period had to be the 1960s. Different cliques wore different styles. There's the Beatles fringe, the sharp Twiggy side part (with the hair like a curtain covering half the forehead), the long Françoise Hardy variety, the asymmetric Peggy Moffitt cut, and puffy Brigitte Bardot bangs.

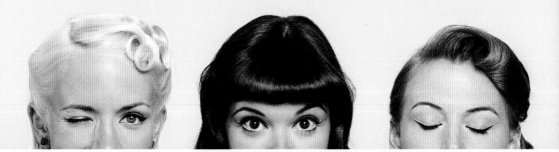

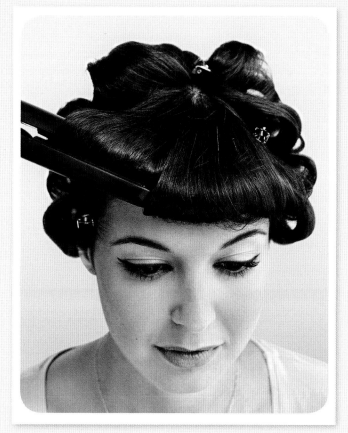

BETTIE BANGS

Inspired by Bettie Page, the rounded Bettie bangs are a true 1950s favorite. A great choice if you're after a playful fringe with an attitude.

HEAT PROTECTANT
CURLING IRON OR FLAT IRON
STYLING BRUSH
HAIR SPRAY

1. Prep the hair with a heat protectant to prevent damage. Part your bangs into three sections, then curl each section inward with a curling iron or flat iron. Let cool.

2. Brush through hair with a styling brush to ensure your hair is smooth and even. Spray the hair with a few thin coats of hair spray.

𝓣ip!

Brush your hair lightly to the side to quickly transform your Bettie bangs into an Audrey fringe!

FAUX BETTIE BANGS

Achieve great fake bangs by simply rolling up your long hair. Perfect when you're looking for a little variation and want to play around with bangs—without losing your locks.

FOAM ROLLER OR OTHER FILLER
BOBBY PINS
HAIR SPRAY

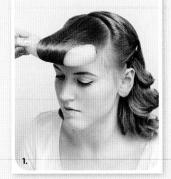

1.

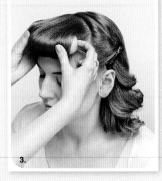

3.

1. Gather a triangular section of hair around the forehead. Roll the hair up on the foam roller. Start with the very ends and roll all the way in toward the head.

3. Distribute the hair evenly over the foam roller to make sure it's entirely covered (you'll be leaving the roller in).

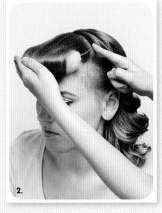

2.

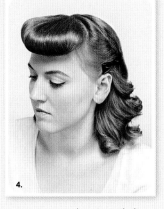

4.

2. Fold in the ends of the foam roller, then fasten it close to the scalp with bobby pins.

4. Once you're happy with the result, spray to set the style.

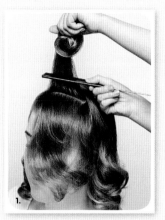

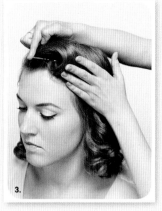

Roll up your hair into a side roll for a playful and elegant take on bangs. You'll need at least medium short hair for this style.

You'll need

TAIL COMB
BOBBY PINS
HAIR SPRAY

1. Pull your bangs sideways in your preferred direction. Comb through the bangs with a tail comb before lifting them up and away from your face as you gently tease the hair.

3. Gently lift the hair off your fingers and keep the roll in your cupped hand. Set the style by securing a few bobby pins inside, as close to the scalp as you can get. Set with hair spray.

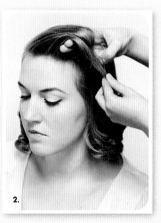

2. Roll up your bangs on two or three fingers. Use your right hand as a "spool" for bangs to slant to the left and vice versa for the right. Roll the hair toward your forehead so that the roll rests inward. Keep rolling the entire section of hair and fold in the ends.

SIDE TWIRL

Looking to create a deluxe everyday hairstyle? Twist your hair into a side twirl—super easy and strikingly gorgeous. Perfect if you have at least medium-length bangs.

You'll need

CURLING IRON OR FLAT IRON
TAIL COMB
BOBBY PINS
HAIR SPRAY

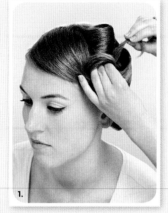

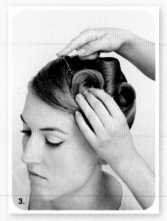

1. Make a side part and gather a fairly large section of hair from the side with more hair. Curl hair ends from that section with a curling or flat iron to achieve a smooth curl (it is much easier to work with curly hair than straight).

3. Gently lift the curl off your fingers and make sure the hair ends are under the curl, toward the scalp. "Lock" the roll in place by pinning it with bobby pins that you secure from the top down.

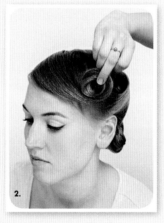

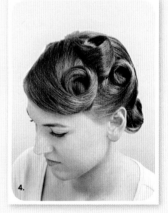

2. Comb your bangs down and a little to the side using a tail comb. Then roll the hair up on two fingers—clockwise for bangs on the left side of your face and counterclockwise for right-side bangs.

4. Spray to set the style.

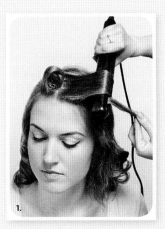

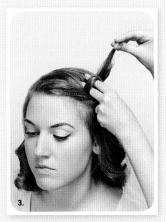

LOOP HAIRSTYLE

Get in the loop! Create an elegant and quick 'do in just a moment. All you need is a tail comb, a curling iron, hair spray, and a few bobby pins.

1. Prep the hair with a heat protectant to prevent damage. Use a tail comb to gather a section of hair around the fore-head about 2 in/5 cm wide. Use a curling iron or flat iron to lightly curl the hair to make it more manageable.

3. Wind the hair up on two fingers in an upward direction (see Victory Rolls, page 60). Don't roll in the tip of the hair. Instead, wind it in the oppo-site direction of the loop and secure with pins.

You'll need

HEAT PROTECTANT
TAIL COMB
CURLING IRON OR FLAT IRON
BOBBY PINS
HAIR SPRAY

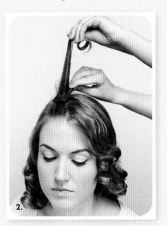

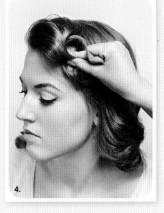

2. Tease the hair closest to the scalp to create more volume.

4. Push the loop toward your part and secure with bobby pins. Spray to set the style.

45

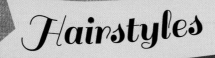

Hairstyles

Get the Look

FANCY CLOTHING IS ALL VERY FINE, BUT NOTHING COMPARES TO A BEAUTIFUL HAIRSTYLE TO TOP IT OFF. A TRUE COMPLIMENT GENERATOR! ROLL UP, COMB DOWN, AND CREATE A NEW LOOK IN JUST A FEW MINUTES. ALL YOU NEED IS THE WORLD'S LEAST EXPENSIVE BUT MOST BRILLIANT ACCESSORY: YOUR HAIR.

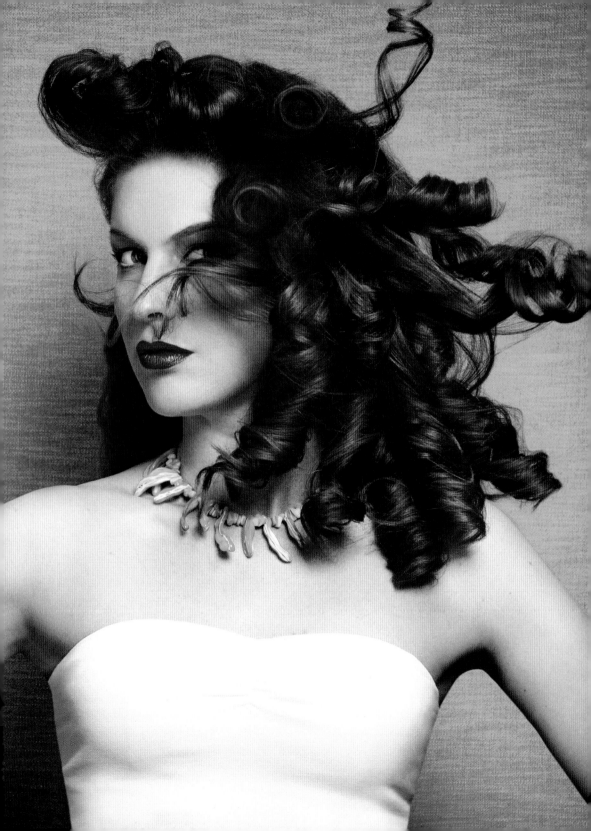

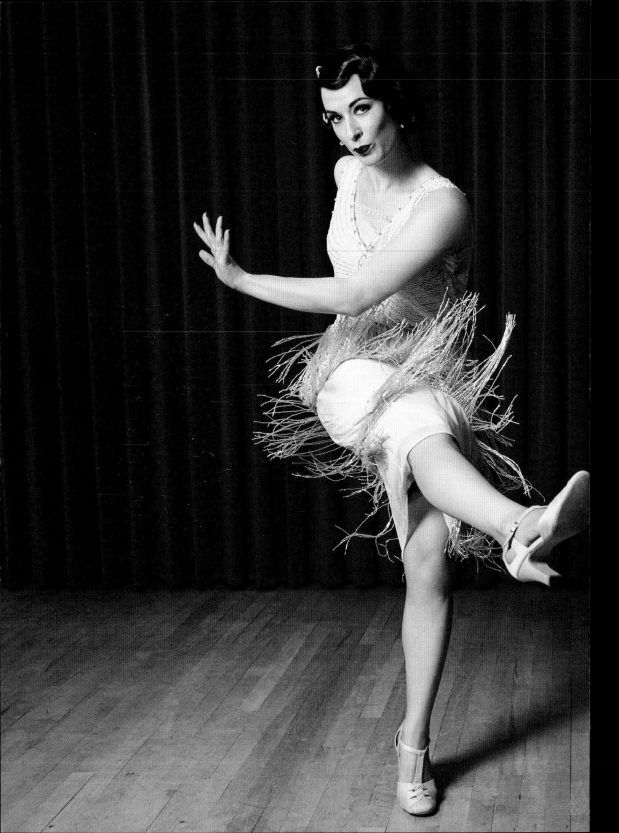

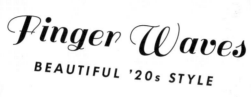

Finger Waves

BEAUTIFUL '20s STYLE

FINGER WAVES

Elegant and groundbreaking, the hairstyles of the '20s sent shock waves through society back in the day. Now this style is the epitome of refined elegance. Find your daring 'do.

You'll need

HAIR GEL
TAIL COMB
WAVE CLIPS
HAIR SPRAY

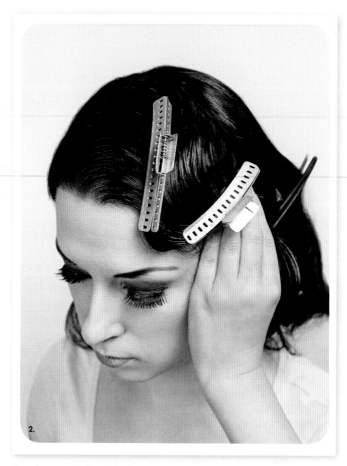

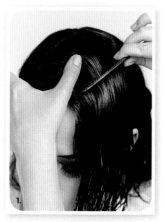

1. Start by soaking the hair (the wetter the better), then prep it with liquid hair gel. Make a sharp side part using a tail comb and then comb all the hair straight down. Gently push the hair up toward your part to see which direction your hair prefers. Then follow that direction by combing the hair in C-formed shapes. Add pressure with your thumb to keep the combed part of the wave in place.

2. Keep the first wave in place with two to three fingers and then start combing horizontally in the opposite direction. Work the waves in a zigzag pattern. Once you're happy with the number of waves, add pressure with the palm of your hand to get more defined waves.

3. Secure each wave with wave clips, fastening where the wave is about to change direction. Let hair set with clips until it is thoroughly dry. Remove the clips and carefully comb the waves. Set the style with hair spray and put the clips back in place while the spray dries. Once dry, remove the clips and your style is done.

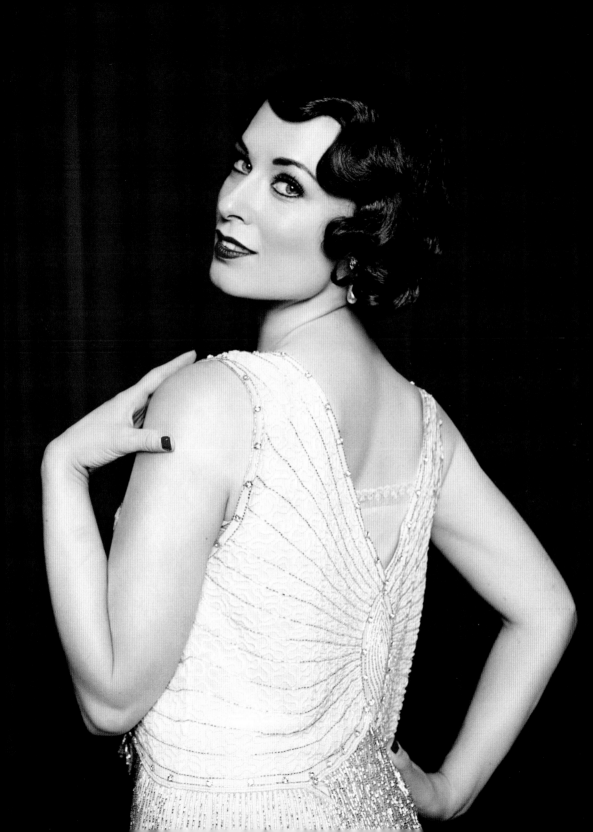

LARGE BILLOWING WAVES

You'll need

MOUSSE OR SETTING LOTION
TAIL COMB
CURLING IRON OR ROLLERS
WAVE CLIPS
STYLING BRUSH
HAIR SPRAY

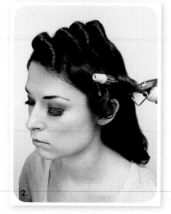

2. Curl the side hair in the same way, but aim to position curls at a diagonal angle.

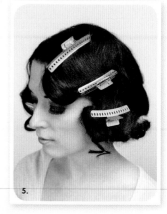

5. Spray to set the style. Before the spray dries, put wave clips in the spot where the waves change direction. Use the clip to pinch up some height in the wave.

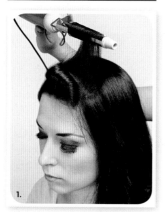

1. Prep the hair with mousse or setting lotion. Use a comb to create a side part, then, using a curling iron or rollers, curl dry hair, making sure you curl all the hair in the same direction—either forward or backward. Try to make all the curls the same size. Remove each curl from the curling iron or roller, roll it up on your finger, and secure with a clip. Make vertical curls along your part.

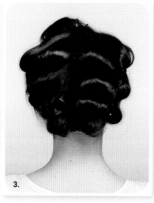

3. As you reach the back of the head, you can curl in two ways: either horizontally for less wave but more volume or vertically for more defined waves but less volume.

4. Once the curls have cooled, remove the clips and brush the curls gently straight down. Using the palms of your hands, push to define waves up toward the part.

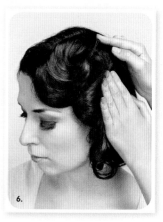

6. When the spray is dry, remove the clips. Secure bobby pins at the center of a wave if you'd like it to be more defined. Mist the hair with a few more thin coats of hair spray for shine and lasting hold.

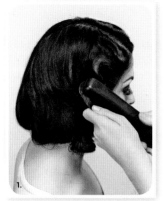

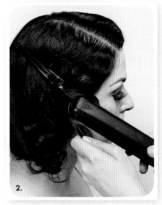

You'll need

HEAT PROTECTANT
SETTING LOTION
FLAT IRON
WAVE CLIPS
COMB
HAIR SPRAY

1. Prep the hair with a heat protectant and setting lotion and make sure the hair is dry before you start. Gather a section of hair roughly the same width as the tongs of your flat iron. Gently push the hair up toward your part to see which direction your hair prefers. Keep pushing the hair up to form a C-shape. Use the iron to flatten the C-shape. Don't pull the flat iron along the hair. Instead, use it to simply pat the hair lightly between the tongs a few times. After this first C-shape, push the hair upward again—this time in the opposite direction. Pat the new C with the flat iron a few times. Once this C is set, push the hair upward again to form yet another C. Keep working in this way all the way down—alternately going left and right—until you reach the tips of the hair.

2. Let the wave cool off, then secure it with a wave clip to keep it out of the way while you work your way through the rest of the hair. Let a thin section of the already waved hair hang loose and use it as a template. Now repeat the wave-making, mimicking the shape of the template all the way to the tips. Repeat with the desired number of sections (2 to 3 usually go a long way).

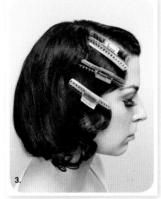

3. Once the waves have cooled off, comb them out into a single wave. Spray to set the style, then attach clips at every point where the waves change direction. Once the spray has dried, remove the clips.

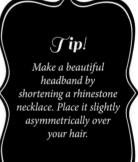

Tip!

Make a beautiful headband by shortening a rhinestone necklace. Place it slightly asymmetrically over your hair.

STARLET'S CURLS

Cheeky and sensual at the same time, this 1930s style is sheer confidence, bottled up.

You'll need

HEAT PROTECTANT
HOT STICKS OR FOAM ROLLERS
NATURAL BRISTLE BRUSH
TAIL COMB
FLAT IRON
HAIR SPRAY

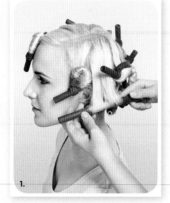

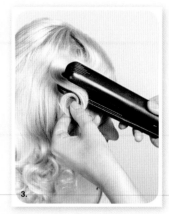

1. Prep the hair with a heat protectant to prevent damage. Roll dry hair on hot sticks. Let cool completely before removing sticks. Always roll hair at the top of the head first. You can also do a wet set on bendy rollers or rags (rag curls) and wait until hair has dried completely.

3. Using the flat iron, make a wave on each side of the face (see Faux Finger Waves, page 53).

4. Lift your curls up on your fingers and mist lightly with hair spray. Layer with several thin coats to increase body.

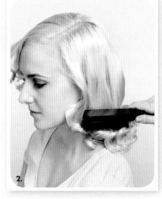

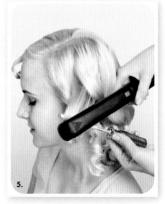

2. Gently brush out the curls with a natural bristle brush to increase body and bounce. Don't brush each curl separately; instead brush them all at once. This style calls for unruly curls. Tease the ends a little with the tail comb to increase volume even more.

5. A different way of achieving this curl is to roll hair on a metal tool you have on hand, like a screwdriver. Once hair is rolled onto the metal end of the screwdriver or other tool, keeping the tool in place, use a flat iron to flatten repeatedly from different directions. Remove hair from the tool and brush lightly.

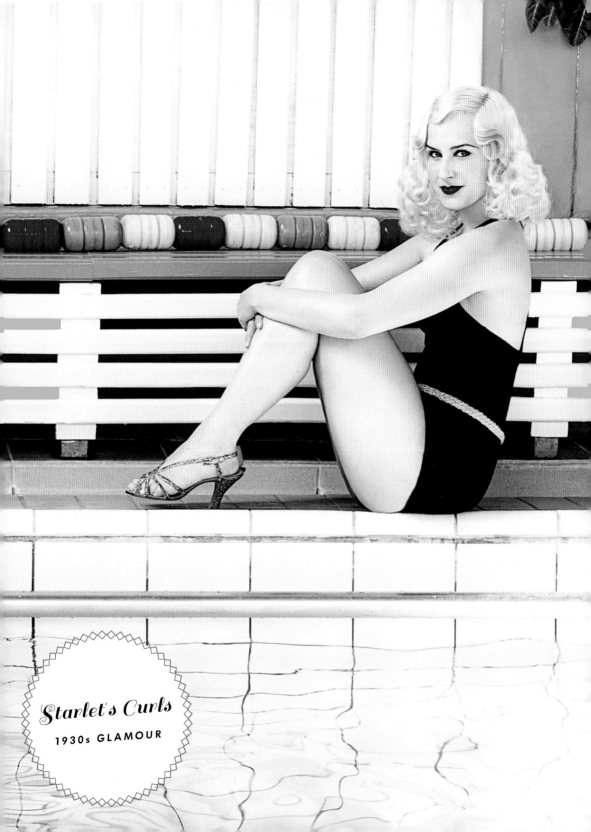

Starlet's Curls

1930s GLAMOUR

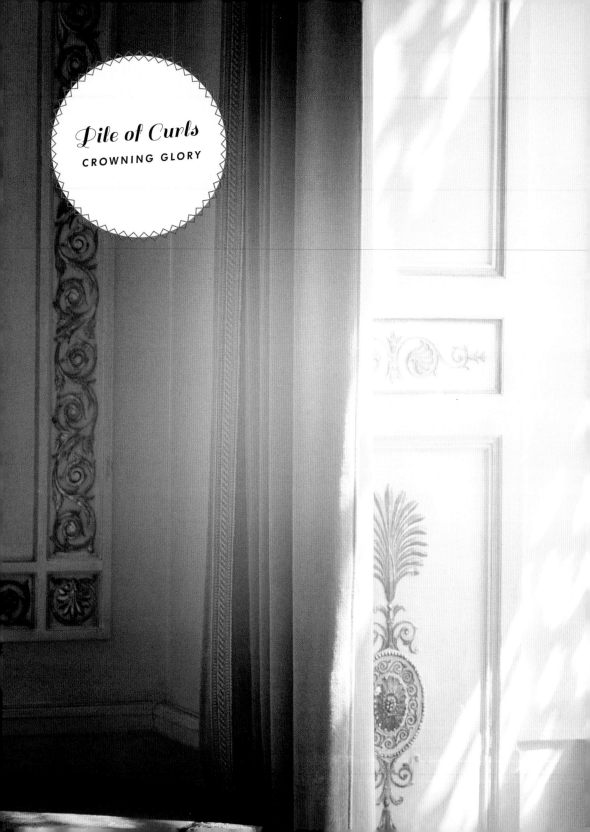

Pile of Curls

CROWNING GLORY

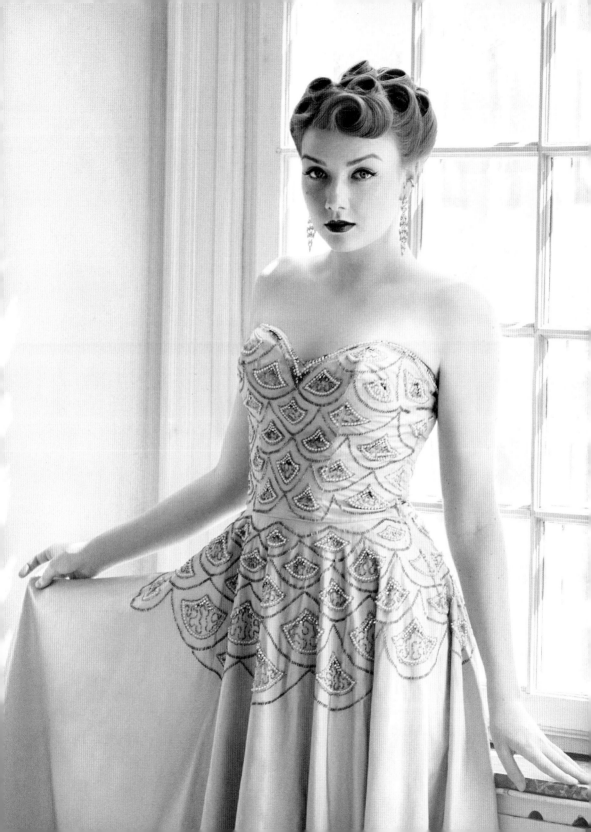

PILE OF CURLS

The idea is simple—just pile on the curls—but this hairstyle looks very complicated: impressive, eye-catching, and supremely stylish.

You'll
need

HEAT PROTECTANT
CURLING OR FLAT IRON
TAIL COMB
LARGE HAIR CLIPS
BOBBY PINS
DECORATIVE HAIR CLIP (OPTIONAL)
HAIR SPRAY

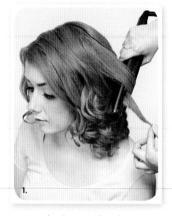

1.

1. Prep the hair with a heat protectant to prevent damage. Curl your hair inward (toward your face) with a curling iron or flat iron (see pages 32 and 33).

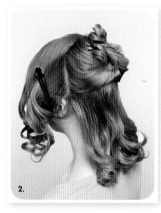

2.

2. Use a tail comb to part the hair from ear to ear across the top of your head, creating two sections, front and back. Pull the front hair forward and secure on each side with large clips. This will keep the front sections out of the way while you're working with the hair in the back. Now divide the hair on the back of the head into an upper and a lower section using the tail comb. Lift the upper section forward toward the face and tuck it out of the way with a clip.

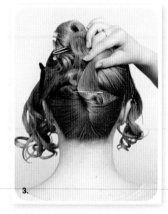

3.

3. Brush the lower section upward and gather the hair into a tail that you twist one turn, then secure two or more bobby pins across the twist (at least one from each direction). Crossing bobby pins "locks" them in place, making the end result more stable. Make sure the bobby pins are fastened tightly and close to the scalp. Instead of using bobby pins, you could also use a stylish hair clip across the twist.

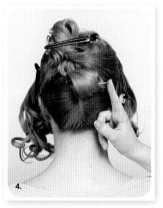

4.

4. Take hold of the top of the twisted section and roll it into a loop about two fingers thick. Place the loop directly on top of the crossed bobby pins to hide them. Pin one or more bobby pins into the loop to secure it.

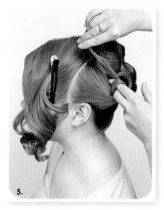

5.

5. Remove the clips from the upper section of the hair on the back of the head. Divide it into smaller sections. If you gather the hair diagonally, your partitions will be less visible in the final 'do.

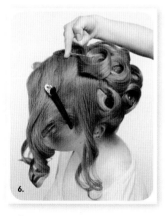

6.

6. If you'd like more volume, tease each section a bit before you curl it. Then wind it into loops by wrapping the hair around two fingers. Place the loop where there is room and it looks best. Alternate winding up on your left and your right hand. Gently lift the loops off your fingers and make sure the tips are placed against the head, between the scalp and the curl, at the base of the loop. Let the loop stand

up like a cylinder and secure by pinning it down inside the loop towards the scalp with bobby pins.

7. Remove the clips from the side hair, which has until now been tucked away. Brush lightly, then divide into smaller sections.

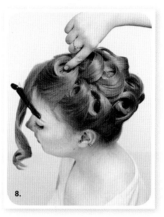

8.

8. Work according to the techniques for Victory Rolls (page 60). Wind loops onto two fingers, clockwise on your left side and counterclockwise on your right. Then gently remove the loop from your fingers and wind the last part of the section into the loop. When the loop is finished, tip it toward the back. Secure it in place with one or two bobby pins at the top of the loop. Try to push the pins in a bit to make them less visible.

9. The bangs (see photo, page 57) are treated like a Side Roll (page 43).

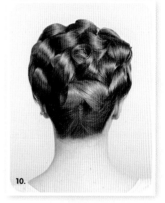

10.

10. To set the style, mist hair with several thin coats of hair spray, which increases hold.

> *Tip!*
>
> *Making a pile of curls is a bit like assembling a jigsaw puzzle. If you're not happy with the hairstyle, there's no need to let all the hair down. Simply remove pins from the loop you don't love and redo it or change the direction of the curl.*

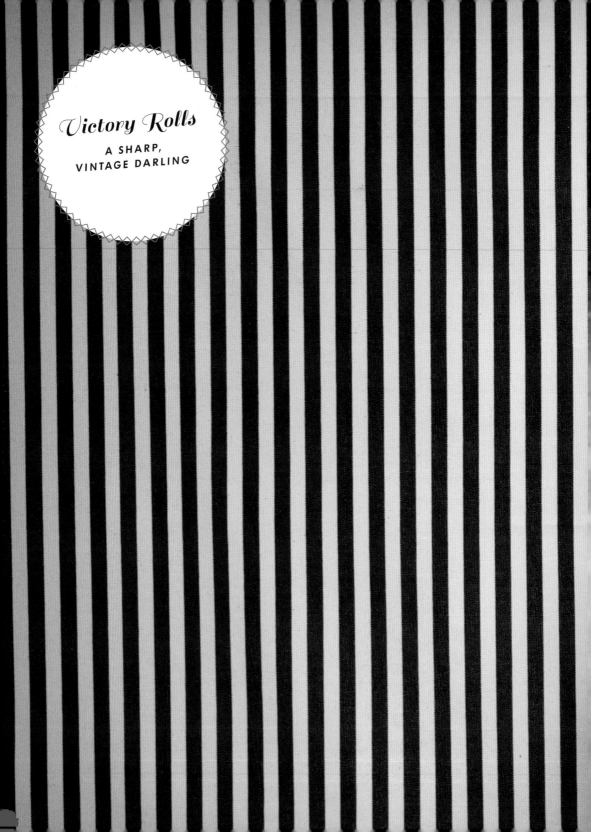

Victory Rolls

A SHARP,
VINTAGE DARLING

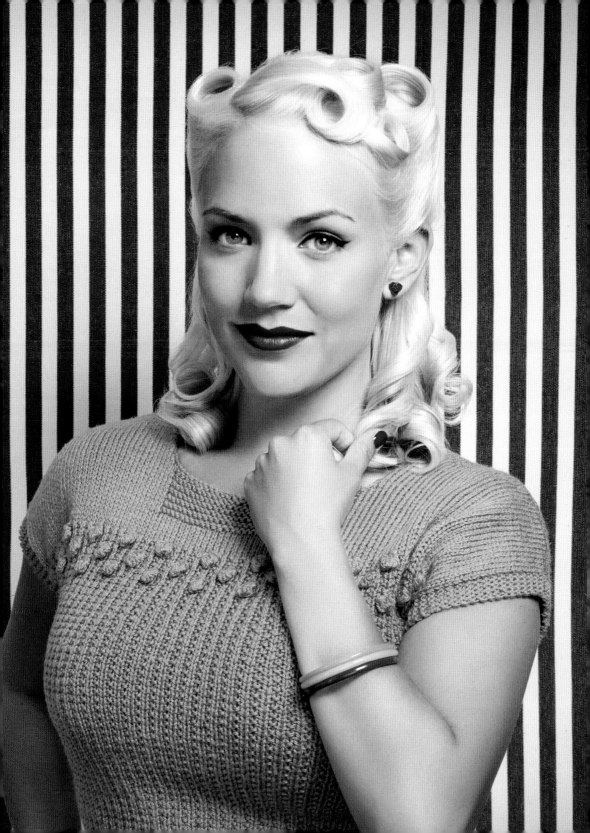

VICTORY ROLLS

Roll your hair into the most winning style of the twentieth century.

You'll need

CURLING IRON OR FLAT IRON
TAIL COMB
BOBBY PINS
HAIR SPRAY

1. To make hair more manageable, curl tips inward with a curling iron or flat iron (see pages 32 and 33). Use a tail comb to gather the section of hair from above your ear to your part. To increase volume, lightly tease the hair close to the scalp.

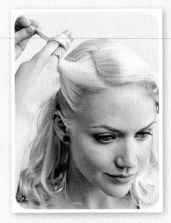

2. Wind the section around two fingers, clockwise on your left side and counterclockwise on the right. If you are right-handed it's usually easier letting your right hand act as a spool and vice versa.

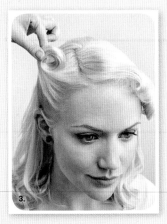

3. Gently lift the hair off the fingers and roll the last little bit of the loop in toward the head.

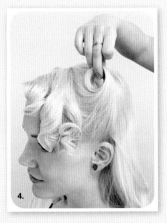

4. Tip the loop toward the back, making sure that the hair tips are tucked in under the base of the loop so they don't show.

Tip!

For a playful take on this iconic vintage hairstyle, divide each side section in two, then make two loops on either side.

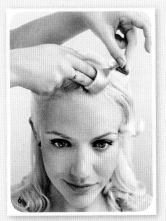

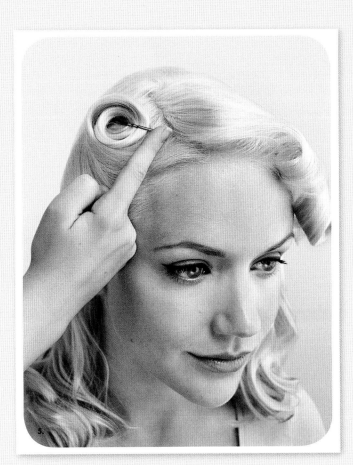

6. Style bangs any way you like (see page 40 for inspiration). In the picture on page 61, we've styled the bangs with one downward loop and two upward. To create the upward loops, treat them just like victory rolls. The downward loop is rolled in the opposite direction—clockwise on the right side and counterclockwise on the left. Pin inside the loops.

7. Spray to set the style.

5. Secure the top part of the loop with one or two bobby pins, pushed in a bit, so that the pin is partially hidden. Push the bobby pin through the front part of the loop but only through half of the thickness of the back part of the loop. This way, the back part of the loop stays a little loose, increasing the volume of the hairstyle.

Poodle with Sweep-Up
CONFIDENT CURLS

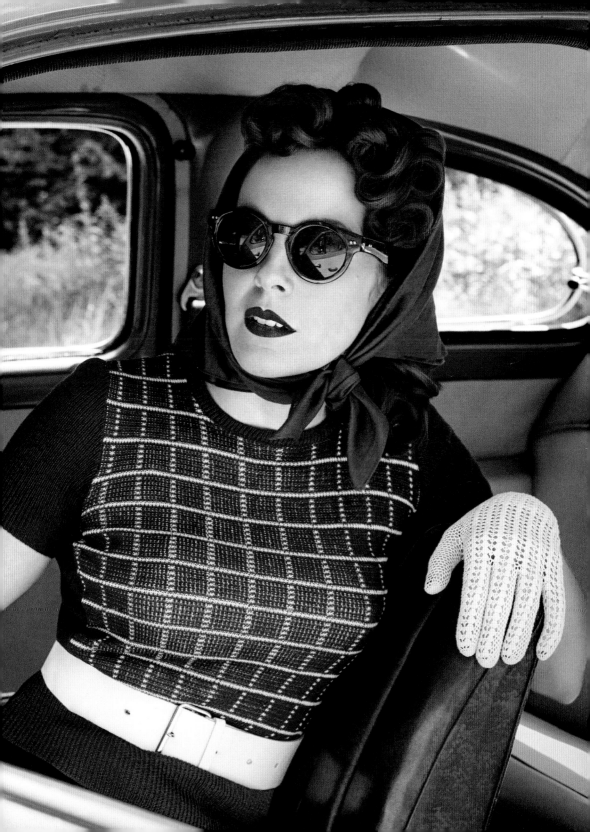

POODLE WITH SWEEP-UP

Bold and beautiful in true Lucille Ball fashion. The poodle 'do is beaming with independence and the spirit of rock 'n' roll.

You'll need

MOUSSE OR SETTING LOTION
SMALL-BARREL CURLING IRON
OR SMALL CURLERS
HAIR CLIPS
HAIR COMBS
BOBBY PINS
HAIR SPRAY

Tip!

This style looks great with a scarf headband. See page 93 for inspiration.

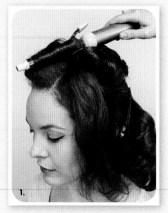

1. Prep the hair with mousse or setting lotion and make sure the hair is completely dry before you start curling. Use a small-barrel iron or roll wet hair on small curlers. Hold the iron under the hair, not over. Curl the whole front section in the same direction, either going left or right.

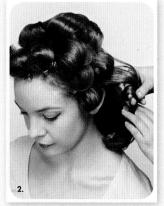

2. Hold until the heat from the curling iron has reached all the way through. Gently open the curling iron a few times to let the curl loose. Roll the curl up on your fingers to prevent it from losing its shape.

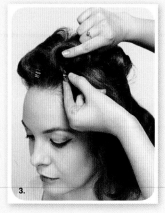

3. Secure by placing a clip at the base of the curl. Let cool.

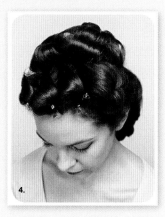

4. Curl the rest of the hair in the same way. When you reach the back section, curl it away from the face, while curling the side hair downward. Follow the same instructions if using curlers, but be sure to wait until hair is completely dry before removing them, and then continue as described on the next page.

5. Once the hair has cooled completely, remove the clips (or the rollers once the hair is dry). Pull your fingers through the hair to separate the curls.

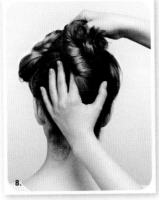

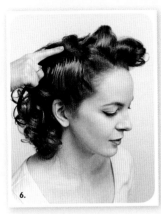

8. To turn this into a full updo—a so-called sweep-up—gather all the hair at the nape of your neck, brush it lightly, and then twist it one turn.

6. Gather the hair high up on each side of your face and secure with hair combs. To secure each comb in place, first comb upward, then push back down.

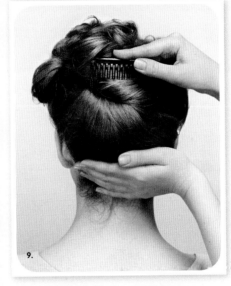

7. Bunch the curls together and secure with bobby pins (be sure not to squish them too much). Push the bobby pins in as close to the scalp as possible, then spray to set the style.

9. Push a hair comb down right over the twist and separate the curls above. Reinforce the style with bobby pins if needed. Finish off with a few thin coats of hair spray.

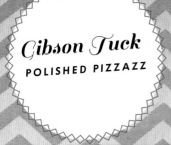

Gibson Tuck

POLISHED PIZZAZZ

1. Prep the hair with a heat protectant to prevent damage. In order to achieve a beautifully smooth roll, start by curling the tips with a curling iron or flat iron. You can make this style on straight or naturally wavy hair, but a little curl helps facilitate the process.

2. Use a tail comb to make a part from ear to ear over the top of the head. Pull the side hair toward the face and hold in place with large clips. Style this hair any way you like (see Victory Rolls on page 60).

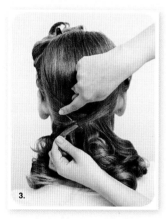

3.

3. Gather a thin section of hair behind each ear. Cross these sections behind the head and secure them with bobby pins at the nape of the neck. This creates a stable base for the style.

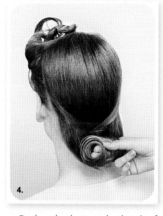

4.

4. Gather the hair at the back of the head together and shape it into one large loop. Use three or four fingers of your right hand as a spool, using your thumb to keep it together. Roll up the loop all the way in to the nape of your neck.

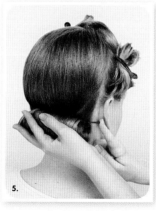

5.

5. Remove your fingers, using your left hand to hold the loop while you pin it in place, securing bobby pins inside the roll. Pinning it high will give it some spring. Use several bobby pins from each direction. You can increase the roll to the width of your choice by gently pulling a bit at the sides.

6. Spray to set the style.

GIBSON TUCK

Gather your hair into a 1940s-inspired roll—a simple and elegant style for both the everyday or a special celebration.

You'll need

HEAT PROTECTANT
CURLING IRON OR FLAT IRON
TAIL COMB
LARGE HAIR CLIPS
BOBBY PINS
HAIR SPRAY

Tip!

For a summery look, attach flowers to the side of the roll. See page 100 for instructions on how to make your own flower clips.

SIDE TWIST

The easiest of all 'dos? The side twist, naturally. Twist, pin, and you're ready to go!

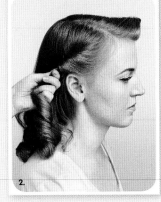

2.

You'll need

TAIL COMB
BOBBY PIN OR HAIR CLIP

2. Twist the hair upward and backward one turn.

1.

1. Use a tail comb to gather the front section of hair on each side of the face, from above the ear to the part.

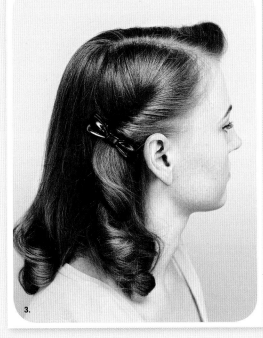

3.

3. Push the twisted hair forward, toward the face. Secure in place with a bobby pin or a stylish hair clip right below the twist.

1. Follow the instructions for steps 1 to 3 for a Gibson Tuck on page 69. Then divide the hair of the back section into three or four parts.

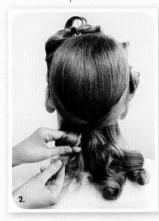

2. Starting from the side, wrap hair around two or three fingers depending on the size roll you want. Use your fingers as a spool to wind up the hair. Wind around the fingers on your left hand to make curls go left or on your right hand for curls to the right.

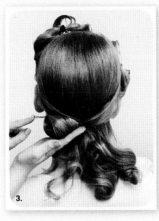

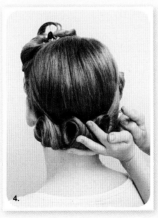

3. As you gently lift the curl off your fingers, make sure the tips of the hair are tucked inside the loop. Then place the loop against the nape of your neck and secure in place with one or more bobby pins fastened inside the loop. Push the pin down from above, at a slight diagonal angle. This way, the pin doesn't show and the loop stays in place.

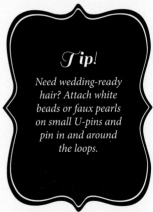

4. Repeat with remaining hair. Roll pieces in the same direction as the previous curl and secure in place closely together. Spray to set the style.

LOW PIN CURLS

Roll your hair into a beautiful party style—it's glamour in three easy steps.

You'll need

HEAT PROTECTANT
CURLING IRON OR FLAT IRON
TAIL COMB
HAIR CLIPS
BOBBY PINS
HAIR SPRAY

Tip!

Need wedding-ready hair? Attach white beads or faux pearls on small U-pins and pin in and around the loops.

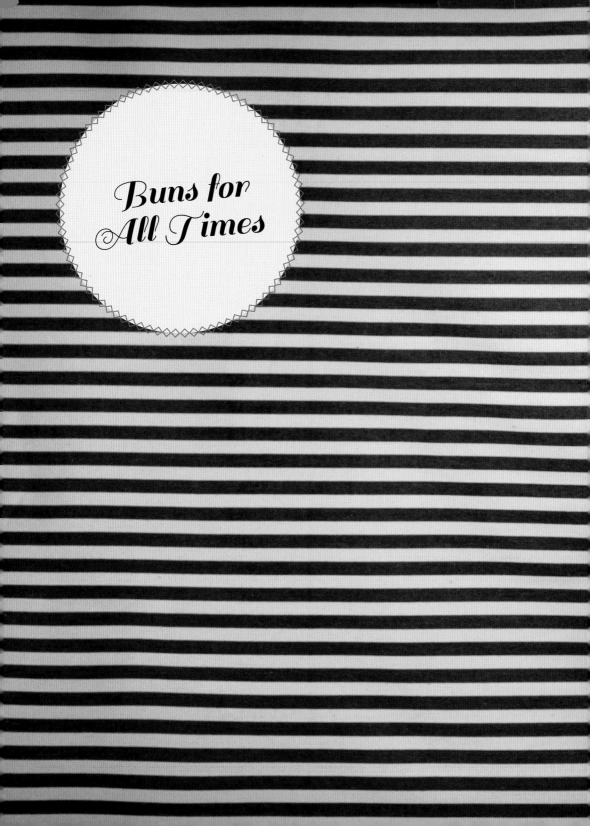

Buns for
All Times

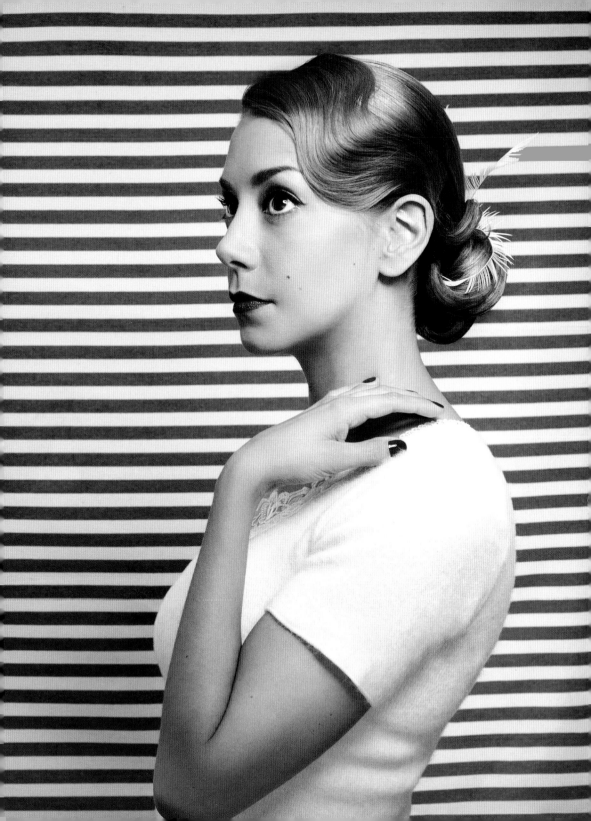

CHIGNON

A regular bun can—with a little extra love—look like an advanced updo. Simply twist and pin and you've got yourself a chignon!

You'll need

HAIR ELASTIC
HAIRNET
BOBBY PINS OR U-PINS

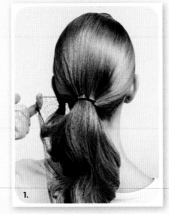

1. Gather the hair into a low ponytail on the middle or side of the head. Cover with a hairnet, which you fasten to the base of the tail with a bobby pin.

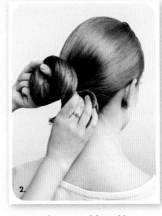

2. Twist the netted hair like a loop. Try turning and twisting in different S-shapes to see which style looks best.

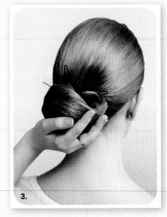

3. Hold the loop in place with one hand and use the other to pin around the edges. You can either use regular bobby pins or U-pins, depending on the texture of the hair. Or use both pin varieties.

4. Decorate the bun any way you'd like; feathers make great accessories. (See page 53 for instructions on the wavy bangs seen on page 73.)

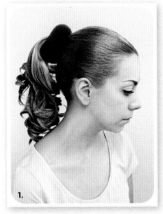

1. Put your hair up in a high ponytail with a hair elastic. Insert hair into a hair donut, then pull the donut close to the head.

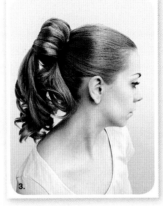

3. Repeat the procedure until all the hair that was in the ponytail is in place around the donut.

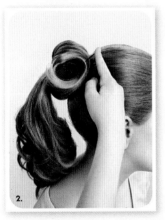

2. Gather a section of hair and bring it in toward the head, around the donut. Secure the hair with a U-pin through the donut.

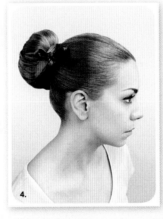

4. Use the last section of hair to wrap around the donut (in the gap between the donut and scalp).

DONUT BUN

You'll need

HAIR ELASTIC
HAIR DONUT
U-PINS

Tip!

Complete the look by tying a silk ribbon around the bun. It makes for a more lavish style and does wonders when it comes to covering up potential flaws.

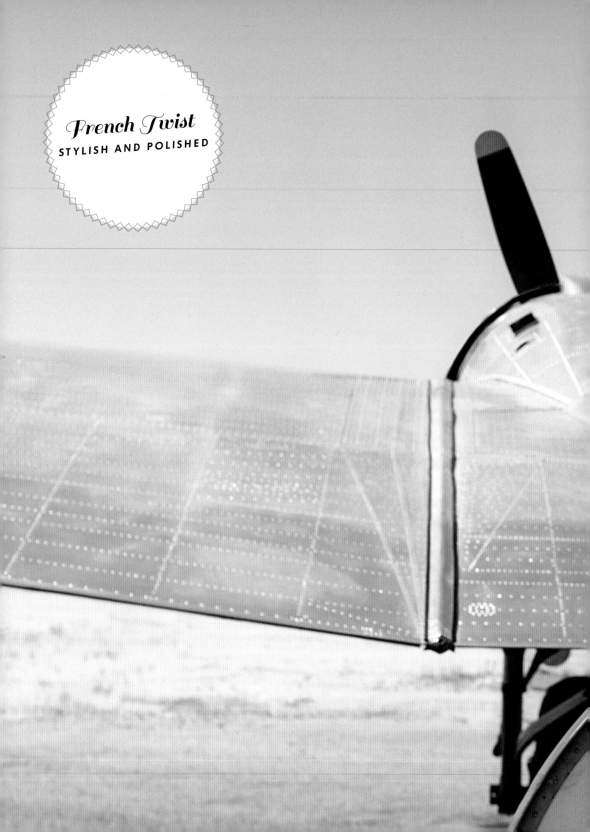

French Twist
STYLISH AND POLISHED

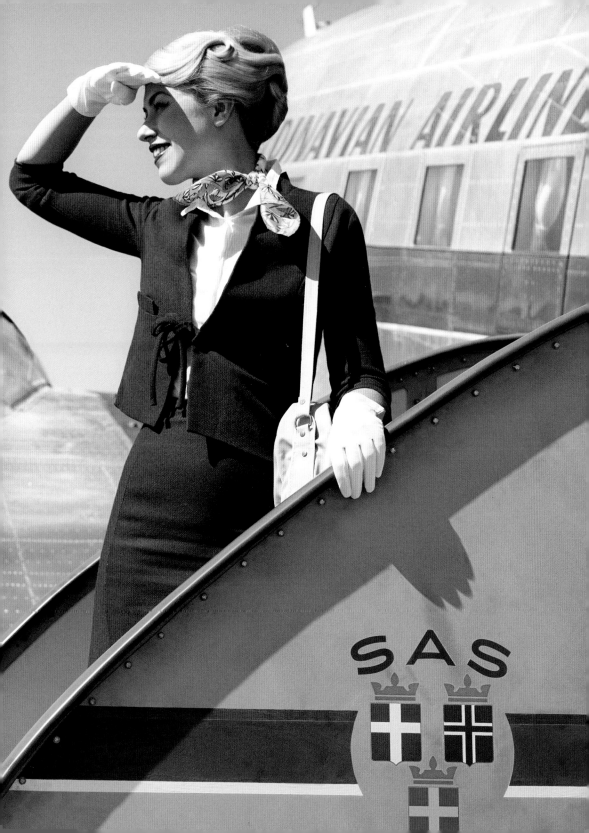

FRENCH TWIST

A timeless classic, displaying both femininity and strength. It doesn't matter if you wear it high or low, as long as you make it your own!

You'll need

HEAT PROTECTANT
CURLING IRON OR FLAT IRON
TAIL COMB
HAIR CLIP
STYLING BRUSH
BOBBY PINS
HAIR SPRAY

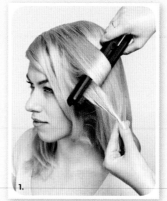

1. To avoid damage, prep hair with a heat protectant. Curl tips inward with a curling iron or flat iron.

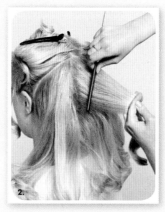

2. Using a tail comb, part the hair from ear to ear across the widest part of your head. Secure the upper section with a clip and start working on the lower section. Tease the hair closest to the scalp in narrow vertical sections. Smooth the surface by gently brushing.

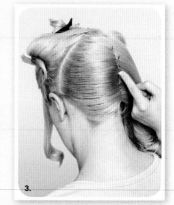

3. Pull all of the hair to one side. Use bobby pins to keep the hair in place on that side. Insert bobby pins in a vertical line, starting from the nape of the neck and working your way up. Overlap the pins a little to avoid gaps.

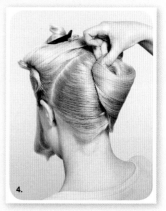

4. Gather the hair and wind it into a cone with the tips tucked into the very center. The cone should have its widest part at the top and the narrowest at the base. Secure the cone by pinning in two places: "inside" in the middle of the cone and along the "edge."

5. Unclip the upper hair and divide into three vertical sections. Start with the middle section, teasing horizontally (from side to side), until you've teased the entire section. Gently brush the surface until smooth.

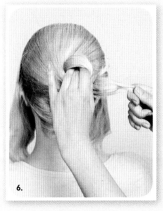

6 & 7. Gather the middle section and wind it into one big loop; tuck the tips inside, toward the scalp. Secure the loop in place above the cone by pinning inside the big loop.

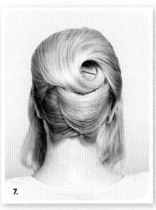

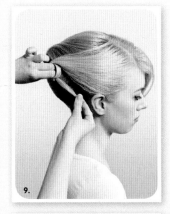

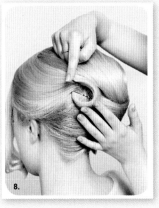

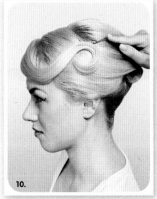

8 & 9. For each side section, gather the hair and wind it into a loop. Turn clockwise on the right side and counterclockwise on the left side. Secure the side loops as close to the back loop as possible, so that the loops form a cluster. Pin just one side of the loop to keep some volume rather than a flat curl. Repeat on the other side. Option: Pin the side loops into the cone.

10. Secure the bangs any way you like. A loop (see Loop Hairstyle, page 45) looks great. Push the bobby pin through half of the loop to fasten it (and make the pin less visible). Spray to set the style.

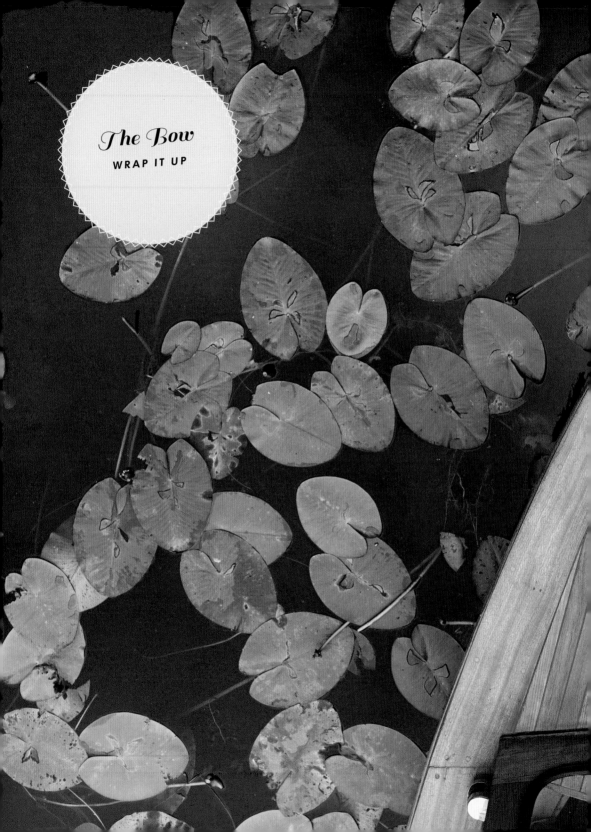

The Bow

WRAP IT UP

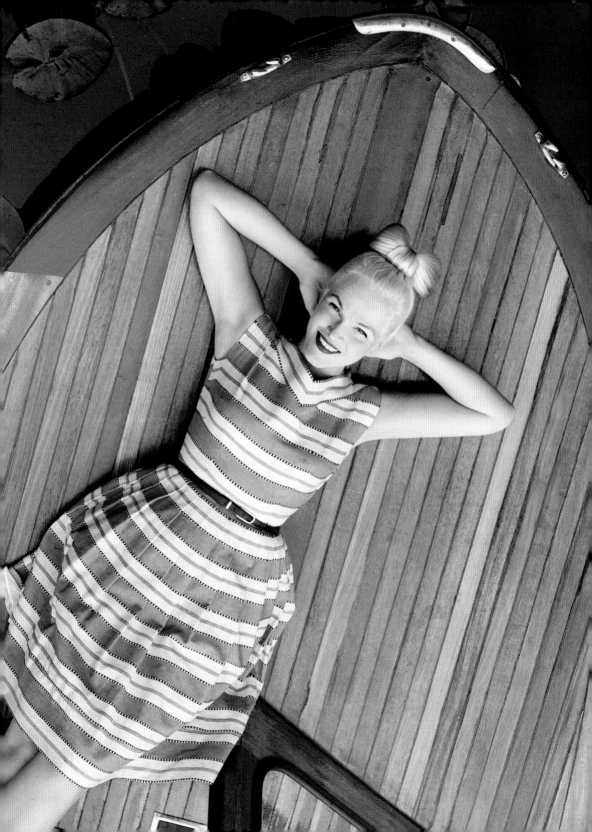

THE BOW

*Don't get tied down to
your usual 'do. Try this
bow instead.*

*You'll
need*

HAIR ELASTIC
HAIR CLIP
BOBBY PINS
HAIR SPRAY

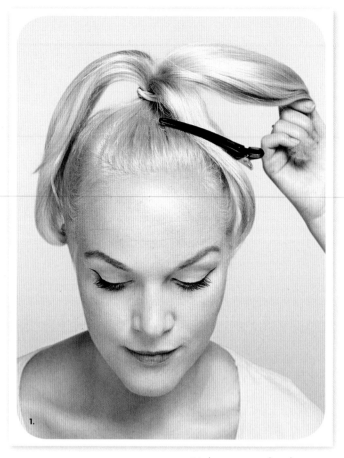

1. Make a ponytail at the top
of your head, as high as possible. Gather a narrow section
from the front of the tail and
secure it out of the way with a
clip. Then divide the remaining
hair into two equal sections.

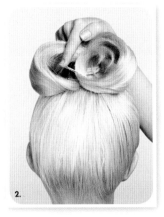

2.

2. Shape each section of hair into a large loop, one in each direction, and fold the tips into the very back of the loop. Secure one side at a time and make sure you push the loops down toward the head to avoid gaps. Fasten with bobby pins as close to the scalp as possible, using a couple of pins for each loop.

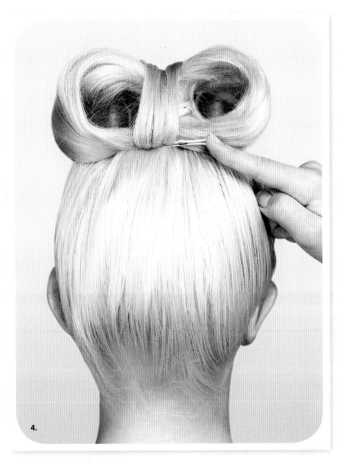

4.

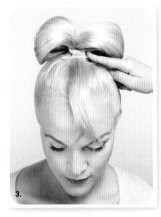

3.

3. Release the section you put aside with a clip. Position the section of hair forward toward the middle of the face. Insert a bobby pin across the section, horizontally and close to the hair elastic.

4. Fold back the hair, placing it right in between the two loops. Secure this section with a pin in the back. Make sure the ends are tucked in. Adjust the middle section of hair and the loops until it looks like a gift-worthy bow. Mist with several thin coats of hair spray to set the style.

THE BEEHIVE

The beehive is a 1960s favorite.
To reach unprecedented heights,
beehive hairstyles were puffed up
with bread loaves and rolls. These
days, there are synthetic fillers and
better hair spray. So enjoy your
bread and keep spraying.

You'll need

HEAT PROTECTANT
FLAT IRON
TAIL COMB
HAIR SPRAY
NATURAL BRISTLE BRUSH
BOBBY PINS

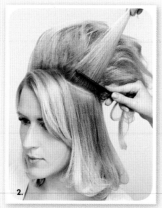

2. Tease the hair, all the way from your bangs to halfway down the back of the neck. Hold each section of hair straight up and tease heavily close to the scalp and more lightly further out. Mist each section with hair spray.

3. Tease the hair on the sides of your head almost all the way down to the ear, holding each section of hair straight up.

5. Gently brush the hair surface with a natural bristle brush. Remember to use a light touch. Part a section of the hair from ear to ear.

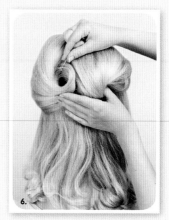

6. Gather half of the back-combed hair and wind the ends into a curl. Secure by placing bobby pins inside the loop and repeat with remaining back-combed hair. You could also just secure the hair in place with a stylish hair clip.

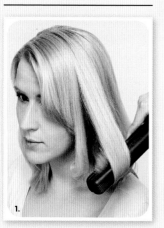

1. To avoid damage, prep the hair with a heat protectant. Curl the tips inward or outward with a flat iron. Inward will make a more vibrant curl, and outward will create a sharp, pointy flip.

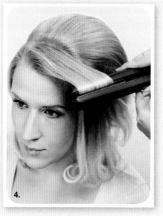

4. With a flat iron, make a bend in the bangs to form a feathered shape by pulling the iron backward and at an angle, while simultaneously rotating it a half-turn inward.

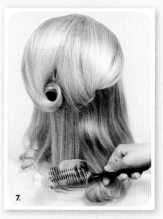

7. Brush the tips outward. Spray to set the style.

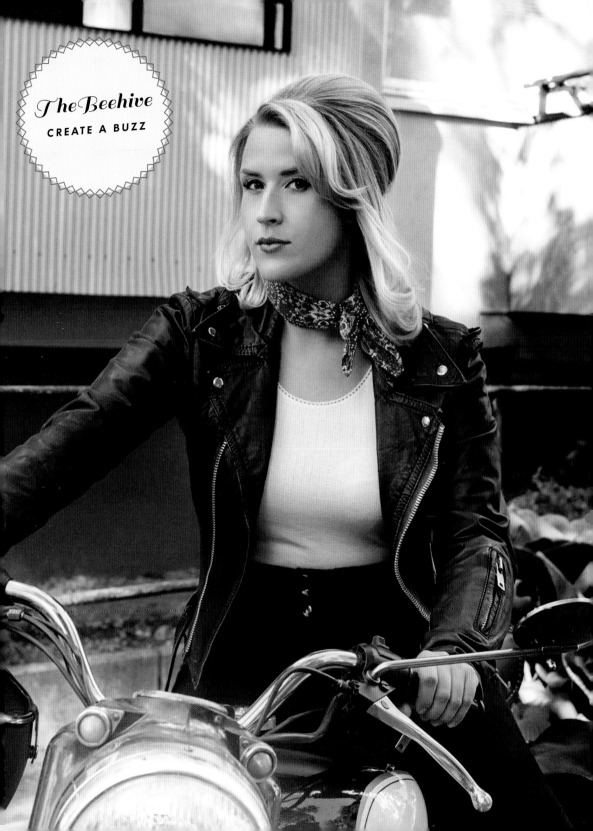

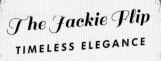

The Jackie Flip
TIMELESS ELEGANCE

1. Prep the hair with a heat protectant. To increase body, stretch the hair straight out on the sides and straight up on the top of the head as you roll it up on a curling iron, flat iron, or hot rollers.

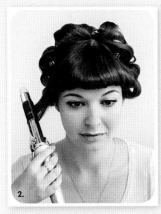

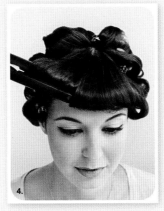

2. The hair on top of the head should be rolled backward, away from the face. All curls should be rolled inward with the exception of the last row of curls, at the nape of the neck; these should be rolled outward.

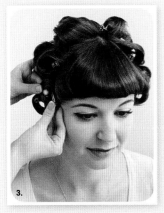

3. Secure each curl in place with a hair clip and let cool. Repeat with remaining sections. (Short on time? Skip this step.)

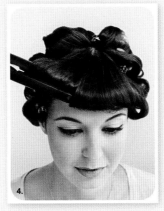

4. Curl bangs in three sections. Start by curling the midsection, then the side sections. This way, you minimize gaps.

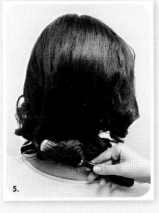

5. When the hair has cooled, let the curls down. Brush all the hair back with a styling brush. Finish by flipping the ends outward.

THE JACKIE FLIP

The immensely popular Jackie flip owes its name to First Lady Jackie Kennedy, who put this 'do on the fashion map.

You'll need

HEAT PROTECTANT
CURLING IRON, FLAT IRON, OR HOT ROLLERS
HAIR CLIPS
STYLING BRUSH
TAIL COMB

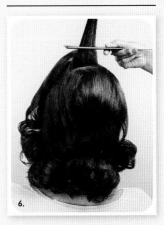

6. Tease the hair on the back of the head in narrow sections, roughly halfway down the back of the neck. Gently brush the surface and spray to set the style by misting the hair with several thin coats of hair spray.

THE BEATNIK'S PONYTAIL

The ponytail swung into glory in the middle of the twentieth century as a symbol of the new teen revolution. Especially sharp when paired with its sidekick Bettie Page bangs, this style is defiant in all its simplicity.

You'll need

HEAT PROTECTANT
CURLING IRON OR FLAT IRON
STYLING BRUSH
BOBBY PINS
HAIR ELASTIC

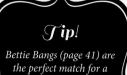

Tip!

Bettie Bangs (page 41) are the perfect match for a ponytail. Part the bangs in a few places so you get a few glimpses of your forehead. Spray thin layers of hair spray to set the style.

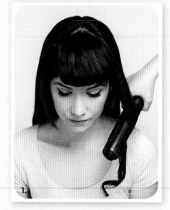

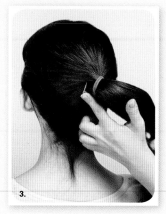

1. Prep the hair with a heat protectant. Use a curling iron or flat iron to curl the hair. Once the curls have cooled, brush through with a styling brush.

3. Push the other bobby pin into the hair, right below the elastic. In this way, you secure the hairdo, resulting in a smoother ponytail.

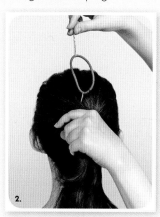

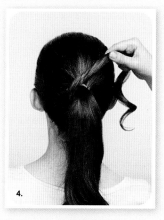

2. Attach two bobby pins on either end of a hair elastic. Brush hair into a high ponytail and grab the tail firmly with your hand. Pin the bobby pin (still attached to the hair elastic) into the upper part of the ponytail, close to the scalp. Wind the hair elastic several times around the ponytail until you can't wind it anymore.

4. Separate a section of hair from your ponytail and wind it around the hair elastic to conceal it. Secure the section back into the tail with an additional bobby pin.

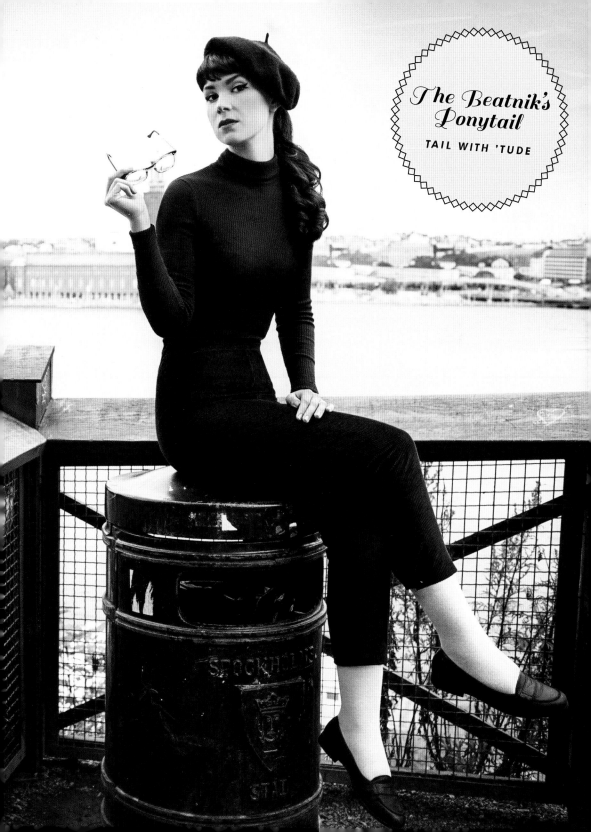

All About Color

FROM A RAVEN-BLACK BOB TO
PLATINUM WAVES, HAIR COLOR
TRENDS COME AND GO.

P latinum blonde, flaming red, or austere black: The urge to change hair color is an ancient desire. Think of the white wig of the eighteenth century; there are many more examples dating back thousands of years. In that time, color-treated hair caught on fire, experienced severe damage, or caused the envy of a whole world. Coloring one's hair has not always been as easy as picking up a package of hair dye in the supermarket or enjoying a salon treatment and a cup of coffee.

For hundreds of years, there has been plenty of experimenting, ranging from mild (such as henna powder made from plants) to wild (such as dubious chemicals). It was not until the early twentieth century that the first synthetic hair color was invented.

In the 1920s, sinful black was the preferred hair shade. This new ideal was a perfect match for the gamine who sent shock waves through Edwardian society by appearance alone. Women used henna to achieve a reddish-brown hue or indigo to create the desired black shade.

As the 1920s turned into the '30s, other colors came into fashion. The movie *Platinum Blonde,* starring an almost white-haired Jean Harlow, opened in 1931 and set the whole world ablaze. Or close to it. Women flocked to hair salons but left with headaches, swollen eyelids, and rashes on their foreheads in order to go blonde. Bleaching was a precise science requiring exact measures of hydrogen peroxide and ammonia—if you messed up, you risked burning the skin. But it hurts to be beautiful, right?

During the rationing times of the 1940s, darker hair came back in style. Ava Gardner and Katharine Hepburn were two major style icons during this era.

After World War II, the dark-haired-woman ideal had worn off. Instead, women yearned to look like blonde bombshell Marilyn Monroe. Platinum blonde hair was suddenly smoking hot. Meanwhile, ad posters blasted out the question, "Is it true . . . blondes have more fun?" The blonde ambition intensified when *Gentlemen Prefer Blondes* hit the screens in 1953. The sequel, *Gentlemen Marry Brunettes,* from 1956 tried to balance the bleached ideal. In the 1950s, hair color as it's now known was launched: Prepackaged, relatively safe, made with chemicals that resulted (hopefully) in the very color displayed on the glossy box.

Spray-on hair color was also a product of this era. In the movies—all in full color now—spray color was used to give both the hairstyle and the color an extra kick. Rumors of this colorized beauty trick traveled fast and far beyond the movie screen. Soon every woman wanted to improve her hair color and look like a Technicolor movie star at the next party.

During the 1960s, flaming red and platinum blonde took a backseat to natural hair colors. The trend was to have truly healthy-looking hair.

Since then, women have continued to change their hair color. In order to realize this dream, strands of hair and sometimes even entire manes were lost in the process—all in the name of beauty. Keep in mind, however, that this was one of all too few ways through which women were able to express their creativity and personality.

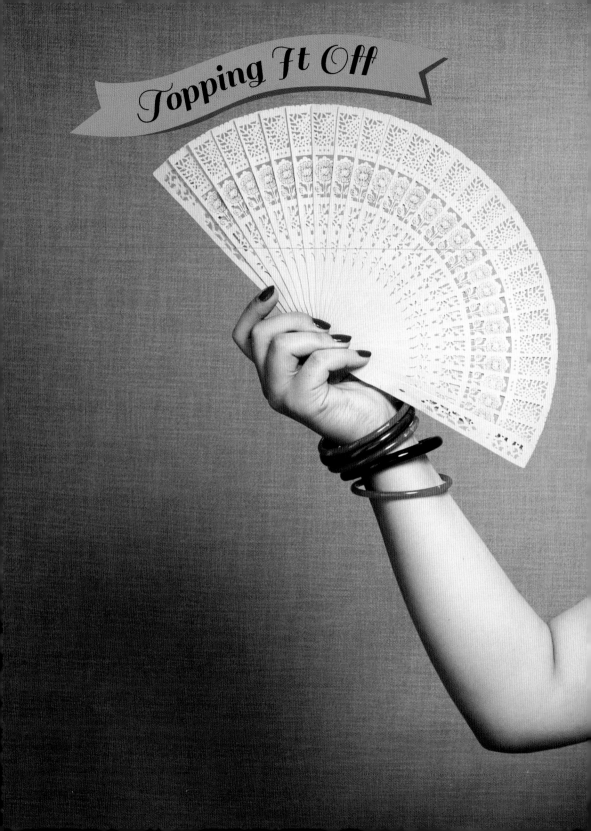

Topping It Off

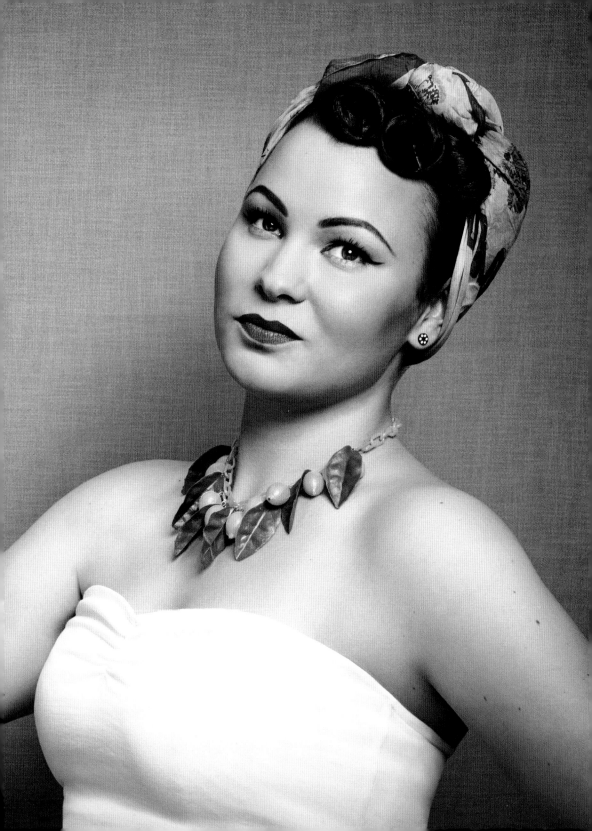

HAT TRENDS

HATS PLAY AN IMPORTANT PART IN THE HISTORY
OF HAIRSTYLES. UNTIL THE '50S, WEARING A HAT
WAS CUSTOMARY, AND LEAVING THE HOUSE
WITHOUT ONE WAS UNTHINKABLE. DURING
THIS HAT-LOVING ERA, HAIRSTYLE FASHION
AND HAT TRENDS WENT HAND IN HAND.

THE 1910s

Around 1910, hats were enormous. The brims were overflowing with feathers, silk flowers, and ribbons. To make sure the hats kept their shape and stayed in place, hat pins were used—in an emergency they could also be used for self-defense purposes. During World War I, hats got smaller and were worn lower and closer to the head (so women who traveled in open cars didn't risk losing their hats). Plumes and delicate decorations adorned the headwear.

THE 1920s

In the 1920s, the hat was pushed farther and farther down and ultimately covered the entire head. The cloche saw the light of day. The brims were small or nonexistent, except for those of summer hats, which doubled as sun visors. Cloche hats and turbans were a great match for the prevailing hairstyle fashions. A few wisps of hair escaping from the trendy bob beneath the hat added a perfect finish to the look.

THE 1930s

During the 1930s, hats shrank even more in size, adorning well-coiffed heads like miniature art pieces. Hats also came in a myriad of inventive, playful, and surreal shapes. Fashion designer Elsa Schiaparelli showcased hats that were true works of art.

Wide-brimmed hats, known as slouch hats, became popular. They paired perfectly with the sensual fashions of the day, and on hot summer days, they doubled as wearable parasols.

THE 1940s

In the 1940s, hats turned adventurous—think Indiana Jones style—and varied in shape. Hats and hairstyles were the best ways to update last year's outfit. There were hats for every face shape and hairstyle. Creating harmony between hair and hat was a way of expressing your style and creativity.

The fedora—worn by both men and women—was a newcomer on the hat scene. Other popular novelties included a version of the bonnet, the halo hat, and the "doll" hat (a small straw hat worn pushed down over the forehead). Once their hat budgets had been spent, many women fashioned new hats out of old garments.

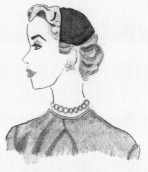

THE 1950s

After World War II, a growing number of women ceased to wear hats on a daily basis. To attract hard-won customers, hats became more varied and lavish. The masculine fedoras were replaced by expressive cartwheels, pancake hats, and turbans.

At home, women protected their curls with headscarves, a tradition from their wage-earning days. Of course, women still worked, but now without a salary.

THE 1960s

Hairstyles grew, grew, and grew. The hat's important standing in previous decades seemed forgotten in the '60s, when enormous beehives ruled supreme. The only hats that had any chance during this era were berets and Jackie Kennedy's famous pillboxes, balancing on top of a big bouffant. From then on, the following rule applied: Hair is the new hat.

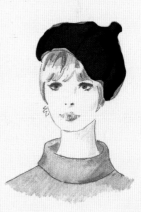

CURL-GUARDING
SCARF MAGIC

Change your look in a flash with a "Rosie the Riveter" scarf, a classic look that dates back to the 1940s. Scarves can be varied infinitely by playing with different tying techniques or fabric patterns. Here's the short list of great scarf styles.

To lure women to the workplace during World War II, the "Rosie the Riveter" campaign was launched all across America. In campaign posters, a strong woman with flexed muscles exclaimed, "We can do it!" Rosie the Riveter became a symbol of female strength, and her look—blue overalls and a headscarf—turned into fashion. In the beginning, scarves were worn in factories for security reasons, but soon enough women realized that scarves were also a great way to protect their curls during long workdays.

TERRIFIC
TURBAN

Protect your curls with a striking scarf style.

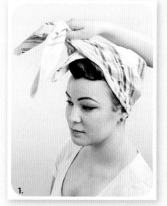

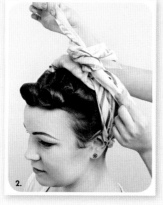

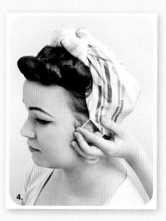

1. Fold a large (27-by-27-in/70-by-70-cm or bigger) scarf into a triangle. Place the scarf on top of your head, letting the middle tip fall down over your nose.

2. Tie the outer tips into a knot. Place the knot on the top middle of your head (to lengthen the look of the face) or slightly asymmetrically on either side (to widen the look of the face). Fold the middle tip under the knot.

3. Make another knot or bow out of the outer tips. If you make a bow, adjust the bow's size until you're happy with it.

4. Fasten the scarf in place with bobby pins. Fold the tips under the sides of the turban, or make a bow out of the tips instead of a second knot. Adjust the bow until you're happy with the size.

CHARMING CONVERTIBLE

Make sure your hair stays in place during windy rides in open cars. Tie a convertible!

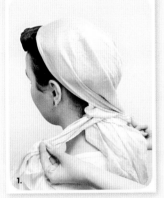

1. Fold a large scarf into a triangle. Place over your head and let the mid tip fall over the back of your neck. Cross the side tips behind your head.

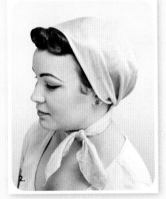

2. Now pull the tips around to the front and tie them into a knot. You can also tie the side tips under your chin without crossing them behind your head.

DECORATIVE HEADBAND

Enhance your style and add a splash of color.

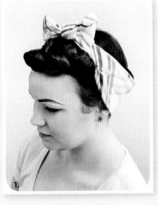

1. Fold a scarf into a triangle. Fold the center tip 2 to 4 in/ 5 to 10 cm inward. Keep folding until the scarf is a wide strip (with the center tip tucked inside).

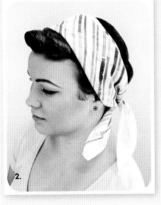

2. Wrap the folded scarf around the base of your neck to your forehead. Choose between tying a knot at the neck or a bow on top of your head. Let the scarf ends hang loose.

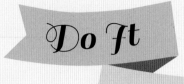

Do It Yourself

MAKE YOUR OWN ACCESSORIES

Pull out plumes, veil fabric, and felt, and put your DIY skills to use as you create your own pretty hats and hair accessories.

PILLBOX HAT

Treat yourself to an elegant Jackie Kennedy hat. It's easy to make, beautiful, and timeless.

You'll need

STURDY FELT FABRIC IN THE COLOR
OF YOUR CHOICE
PEN
MEASURING TAPE
FABRIC SCISSORS
PINS
GLUE
NEEDLE
THREAD
SILK RIBBON

1. Place the felt on a flat surface. Mark out a strip that is roughly 2¾ in/7 cm wide (or as tall as you'd like your hat to be) by 20 to 22 in/50 to 55 cm long (depending on your hat size).

2. Using fabric scissors, cut the felt according to your template, then bring the fabric together to form a circle. Let the ends overlap about 1 in/2.5 cm. Pin the ends together.

3. To create the "lid" for your pillbox, pick a bowl, small plate, or other round object. Make sure the object is the perfect size to fit within your felt circle. Put the round object on top of the felt fabric, trace along the edges, and cut around it.

4. Place the lid over the circle and measure so that it's a perfect fit. Once you're happy with the shape and size, glue the two ends of the circle together. Let dry. Want your hat to last longer? Reinforce it by also sewing the ends together with a few stitches.

5. Add the lid and join the two parts together with a few stitches. Tie a silk ribbon around the hat in a neat bow.

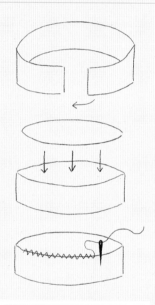

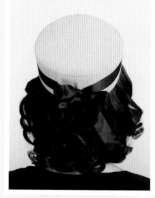

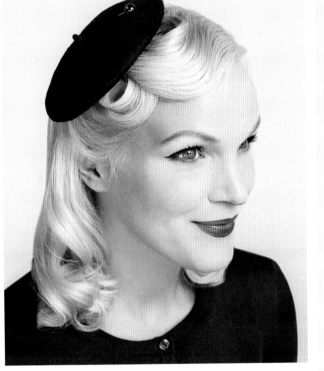

MINI BERET

All due respect to the classic beret, but it doesn't hold a candle to the merry mini beret.

You'll need

FELT FABRIC
PEN
FABRIC SCISSORS
NEEDLE
THREAD
HATPIN

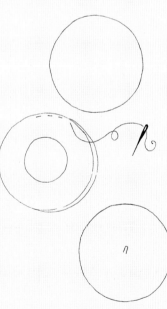

1. To make a template, pick out a round object, like a bowl or plate, the same size you'd like your beret to be. On a flat surface, put the felt fabric on top of your template object. Draw along the edge to make the template. Once you have made a complete circle, remove the object and cut out the template. The pictured beret is roughly 5 in/12 cm in diameter.

2. Repeat step 1 so that you have two identical round pieces. Choose a smaller round object, like a cup, for the bottom of the beret. Place this smaller object in the very center of one of the felt circles,

then draw along the object's edge and cut along the marking.

3. Sew the two pieces together, then turn the whole thing inside out. Your beret is basically done! Press along the seams with an iron if you'd like a flatter beret.

4. Use up some excess fabric by cutting out a ³⁄₁₆-by-⁹⁄₁₆ in/ 0.5-by-1.5 cm piece of fabric. This will make up the beret's "wick." Attach the wick to the center of the beret with a few stitches from the backside. Use a hatpin to secure the beret to your hairstyle.

FLAPPER FINESSE

Turn a brooch into a 1920s-inspired feather accessory. Classy and simple.

You'll need

BROOCH
FEATHERS
SILK RIBBON
HAIR CLIP

1. Open the brooch and insert the ends of the feathers between the pin and the brooch.

2. If you'd like a headband in true 1920s fashion, cut a silk ribbon to the desired length, then attach the brooch to the ribbon.

3. Insert a clip into the brooch and on top of the silk ribbon, then attach the clip to your hair. This way, the weight from the brooch rests on the clip instead of the silk ribbon (which might otherwise be weighed down).

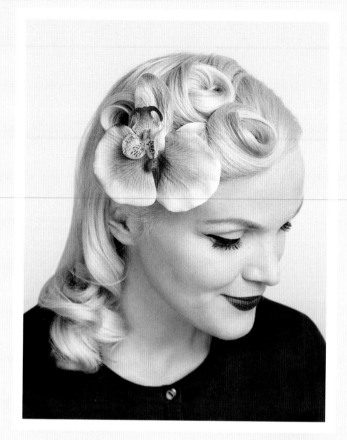

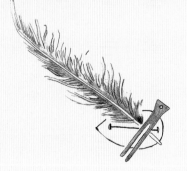

FETCHING FLOWER

The easiest DIY accessory of the century!

You'll need

GLUE
HAIR CLIP
ARTIFICIAL FLOWER

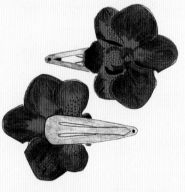

1. Dot some glue on the hair clip, put the flower on top of the glue, and apply light pressure until the flower stays in place. Let dry, and it's ready to wear!

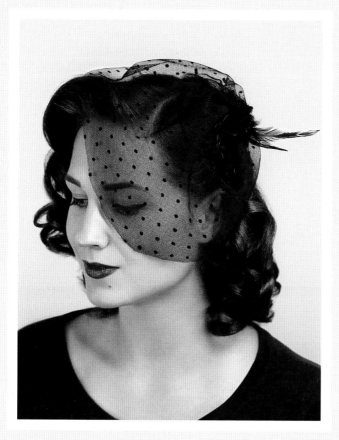

BEAUTIFUL BIRDCAGE

A dramatic and incredibly stylish look for any occasion.

You'll need

SCISSORS
VEIL FABRIC
NEEDLE
THREAD
BOBBY PIN
FEATHERS, PLUMES, SMALL BEADS
HAT BASE
FABRIC GLUE

Tip!

Buy a hat base in a craft store, or make one yourself by coating a round or oval piece of cardboard in felt, or simply use an extra piece of sturdy felt. Attach a hair clip to the felt, and you have a hat base.

1. Cut out a semicircle from the thin, transparent fabric (veil fabric is available in many different varieties). Thread the needle and stitch through the fabric along the straight edge. Once you've stitched all along the edge, gather the fabric together and secure with a pin.

2. Attach feathers, plumes, or small beads with needle and thread, covering the thread ends of the veil.

3. Once you're happy with your arrangement, attach it to a hat base with glue or a needle and thread.

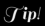

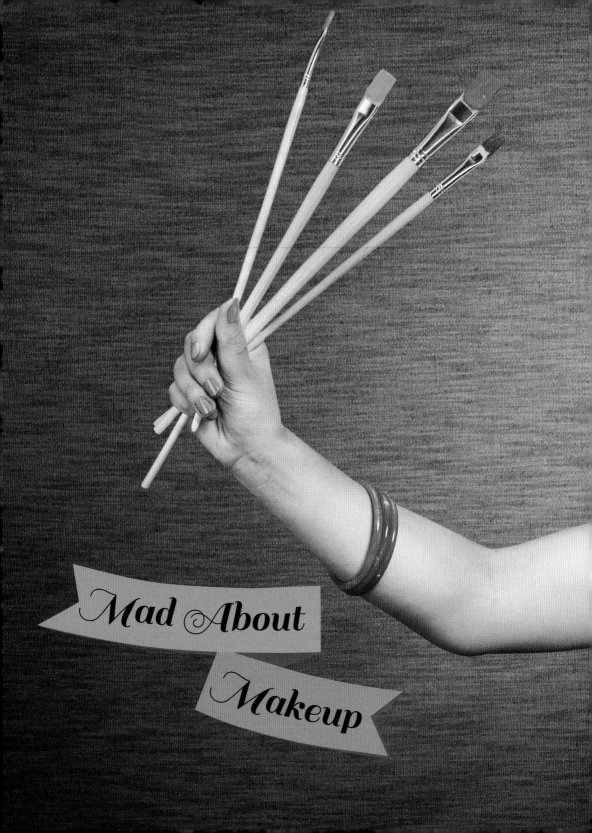

Mad About

Makeup

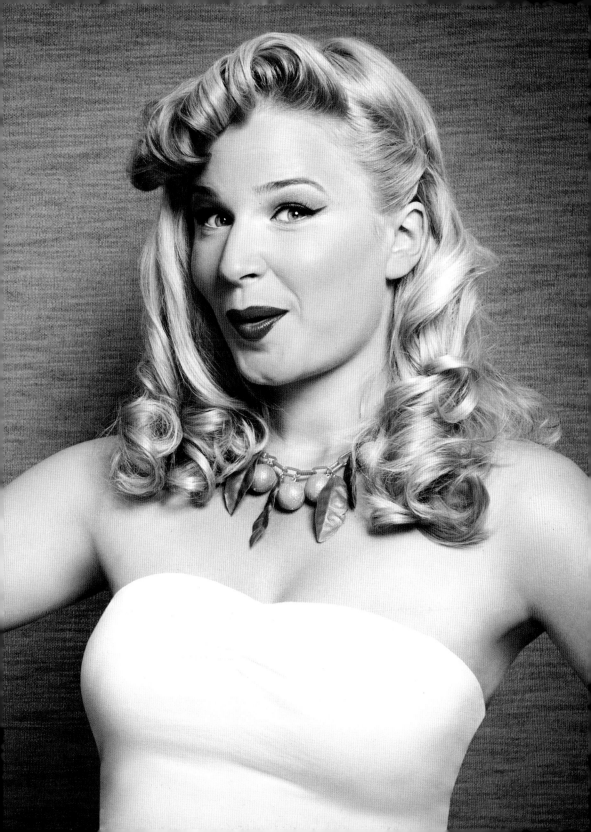

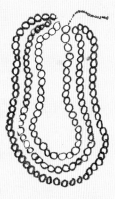

FROM SECRET TABOO TO TRENDSETTING ESSENTIAL

LIPS PAINTED RED, BEDROOM EYES
EMPHASIZED WITH LINER, AND A MEDLEY OF
PASTEL-COLORED EYE SHADOWS: FOR DECADES,
MAKEUP HAS BEEN WOMEN'S MOST EFFECTIVE
WAY OF PROVOKING AND SEDUCING. TOGETHER,
EACH EYELINER WING AND TOUCH OF
BLUSH DRAWS A SHARP COSMETIC LINE
THROUGH HISTORY. JOIN US ON A
POUTY-LIPPED SAFARI THAT WILL TAKE
YOU FROM THE TABOO-RIDDEN 1910S
TO THE TRENDSETTING 1960S.

As movies became increasingly popular in the early
20th century, makeup did, too. Makeup was used to
emphasize contrasting facial features in silent movies.
Eyebrows were painted as sharp lines to underscore facial ex-
pressions, while lips were painted dark red to distinguish them
from pale skin. During this tumultuous period of women's
issues and cropped 'dos, women used makeup to mark their
independence and identity. It was an effective means to alternately please and upset, all while challenging societal norms
and thus breaking new ground. Colors and shapes changed in
step with the advent of color television, new feminine ideals,
and women's budgets.

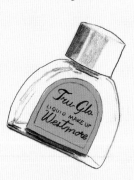

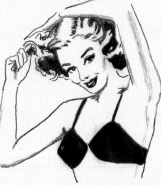

EYES

The birth of mascara; thick, winged eyeliner; and sugar-sweet doll lashes. Learn how eye makeup changed from the discreet 1910s to the pop-arty 1960s.

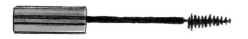

Tip!

Paint your winged eyeliner in three easy steps. Start at the center of the lid and move outward. Then line the corner of your eye toward the center. Finish off with the wing of your choice.

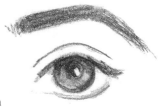

THE 1910s

Up until the 1910s, makeup was used sparingly. To paint one's face was considered taboo. The prevailing ideal was natural, but just as today, "natural" was open to interpretation. Makeup was a well-kept secret, only to be applied when no one was watching. The department store Selfridges in London was among the first to break the taboo when it opened a beauty section, where Brits could buy makeup openly over the counter. Around the same time, Maybelline launched the first mascara, its "cake" mascara, made from petroleum jelly and sooty coal. In Hollywood, movie stars began to paint their eyelids with a paste containing henna extracts, an invention that paved the way for Mr. Max Factor. He soon launched an exciting new product onto the market—eye shadow—in colors like gray, green, and yellow.

THE 1920s

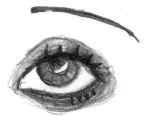

As the 1920s started kicking with the lively Charleston, eyes were painted with dark eye shadow both over and under the eyes. Lashes were darkened with coal dust or with the new cake mascara (which came in a box with mascara, a brush, and a picture of movie star Mildred Davis's eyes). Since the mascara brush was rather flat, women also used a Kurlash eyelash curler. Meeting the demand for expressive eyes, false eyelashes—made from human hair—hit the market. Inspiration for the 1920s look came from the expressive "talking eyes" on the big screen, eyes belonging to newly minted movie stars like Clara Bow.

THE 1930s

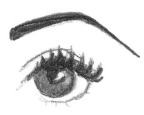

In the 1930s, a more refined look came into fashion. All eyes were on the eyelashes, which were painted with mascara, especially the upper lashes. Lower lashes got just a thin layer or were left as is. Max Factor and Elizabeth Arden were favored brands, on the dressing table, in the handbag, and in magazines. Black-and-white magazines from the 1920s gave way to the lavish color photographs of a new era. The magazines' improved color reproduction paved the way for brightly colored eye shadows.

THE 1940s

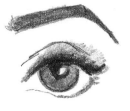

Despite war and rationing, makeup was still an important part of women's everyday life. However, the 1940s were less about expressive eyes than about lips (see page 107). Eyes were painted with light brown eyeliner finished off with a small but distinct wing. Eyelashes were painted with a moderate but sufficient coat of mascara. The look was natural and elegant in all its simplicity.

THE 1950s

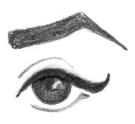

Eyeliner, eyeliner, and more eyeliner: The 1950s were all about eyeliner. It was painted in a thin line along the eyelids with an eyeliner brush and then finished off in a wing. The goal was to create as seductive a look and gaze as possible. Mascara was a girl's best friend, especially if it was the revolutionary new tube mascara from Helena Rubinstein. Lower lashes were left bare. As color movies hit the screens, even lighter, pastel shades of eye shadow, often with a pearly shimmer, became popular.

THE 1960s

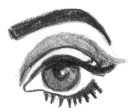

The look of wide-eyed, innocent doll eyes gained popularity during the 1960s. White or light blue eye shadow was painted on lids, before contour lines were painted on with eyeliner. Sprawling spidery lashes were created with coats and coats of mascara (and quite a few false eyelashes) along both upper and lower lids. To underscore the open, wide-awake look, a thick eyeliner line was painted onto the upper lid, white eyeliner under the eye, and, finally, black kohl along the lower lash line.

LIPS

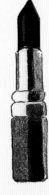

The lip trends of the twentieth century range from small wine-colored lips to pouting Monroe lips to the foundation-treated nude lips of the 1960s. Here's a lip history taking us from women's lib to power lips.

THE 1910s

Giving your lips a healthy touch of color was nothing new, not even around the beginning of the twentieth century. What was new, on the other hand, was the lipstick. This revolutionary essential was invented by Maurice Levy in 1915 and consisted of a colored roll-up stick made out of wax in a metal tube. Lipstick was frequently used by suffragettes and soon came to symbolize female emancipation. Lipstick—or colored lip balm—was applied daintily to the lips.

THE 1920s

During the 1920s, dark red and reddish-brown lipsticks came into use so that lips could be visible on the brand-new silver screen. In order to achieve perfect contours and shapes, lip stencils were used. Lips were painted in a small heart shape, a so-called Cupid's bow. No one even considered following the natural lines of one's lips. The mouth was supposed to be small yet full, a dainty pout in an otherwise pale face.

THE 1930s

The quasi-glamorous yet depressed 1930s left quite a few lip marks behind. Red lipstick was every woman's accessory. The going look was not pouty, but rather square and oblong. Inspiration came from such style icons as Greta Garbo and Marlene Dietrich.

The pale ideal from the 1920s seemed too severe in the already troubled 1930s. Instead, a new sun-kissed beauty ideal came into fashion, adding a golden, sunny shimmer to the reigning superstars. This paved the way for a new kind of product. In the 1930s, the popular brand Helena Rubinstein introduced lipstick with built-in SPF.

THE 1940s

If you think lipstick was not a priority in the midst of a burning war, think again. In America, lipstick was considered a way of boosting morale, a power accessory of sorts. Women were encouraged to wear lipstick to disguise grief, and lipstick became synonymous with strength. With their full, symmetrical lips, Rita Hayworth, Bette Davis, and Joan Crawford were at the forefront of this new trend.

According to the fashionistas of the day, the power lipstick was to be worn together with matching nail polish. Seeing the potential of this concept, beauty brands started offering kits with matching lipstick and nail polish.

THE 1950s

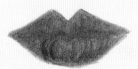

The ultrafeminine fashion characterizing the 1950s was accentuated by pouting lips painted red or pink. The style icons were Marilyn Monroe, with red lips, and Audrey Hepburn, with pink. In order to achieve a fuller look, the lipstick was painted on outside the natural contours of the mouth.

The majority of women wore lipstick all day long. Lipstick was constantly applied and reapplied from tubes in gold-colored cylinders, until chemist Hazel Bishop invented kiss-proof lipstick. This revolutionary product stayed on lips until it was removed.

THE 1960s

To a large degree, this decade was about abandoning conventional takes on beauty. After the excessive lipstick consumption of the 1950s, color seemed to vanish from the lips. Instead, they were painted in pale hues of beige, pink, or white in order to blend in with the rest of the makeup. Nothing was supposed to distract attention from the eyes (see page 106).

Tip!

Start with lip liner, followed by a coat of lipstick. Blot using a tissue, and apply another coat of lipstick before gently blotting again. Matte lipsticks result in a glamorous vintage look!

EYEBROWS

Round, square, full, or nonexistent: Possibly the world's smallest accessory, the brows have played a great part in the history of beauty. From Clara Bow's sharp, inspired lines to Audrey Hepburn's full brows, women expressed their beauty through their eyebrows.

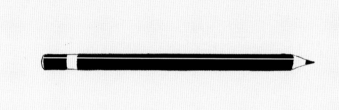

Tip!

Try painting your brows with eye shadow instead of pencil. Use a firm, slanted brush and several short strokes in order to fill in and shape.

THE 1910s

Brows were gently trimmed and shaped with tweezers, and remained relatively natural in shape.

THE 1920s

Short, thin brows were shaped like an arch or a sloping line to create the fashionable, somewhat unhappy look. Brows were drawn on with black or brown eyeliner.

THE 1930s

The thin ideal was still in, but brows stretched farther. Greta Garbo set the trend with her defined long-arched brows. Somewhat thicker brows started to become en vogue. Petroleum jelly or olive oil was applied to increase gloss.

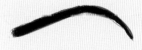

THE 1940s

During the war-stricken 1940s, brows got a makeover. The ideal was a natural look, tweezed to perfection. Both rounded and square shapes were in fashion.

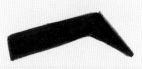

THE 1950s

Brows reached new heights during their golden era of the 1950s. Expressive, full of character, and very thick, they framed eyeliner-enhanced eyes. More was more when it came to makeup, both with shape and color. The heavily arched eye-catching brows were preferably one or several shades darker than one's natural color.

THE 1960s

To some extent, the fuller-brow trend continued well into the 1960s. Brows were tweezed and filled in, just like in the 1950s. But a new distinct trend also saw the light of day—natural-colored, arched, and tapered brows.

BLUSH

A rosy cheek or a promiscuous accessory? Despite its simplicity, this little cosmetic invention managed to create quite some controversy.

THE 1910s

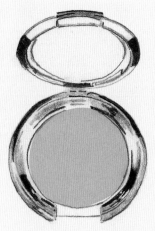

The ideal was to look as fresh as a rose. Pale skin—indicating that you didn't spend a lot of time in the sun—was considered the height of elegance. Max Factor introduced pancake makeup in 1914. Originally made for screen appearances, it resulted in a smooth finish. Fashionistas quickly made it an essential part of their equipment. Around that time, the same brand launched a blush in a practical portable case. On top of the pale skin, light blush was applied with a pad. The ideal was a very natural look. Too much blush and you risked being considered provocative or even promiscuous.

THE 1920s

Many women maintained the pale ideal with a new lead-free powder (up until this point, lead was a popular ingredient). On the powdered, matte cheeks, red or orange blush was applied all the way up to the eyes. Portable blush cases were introduced on the market, helping this makeup novelty become more socially accepted. It was easy to apply, convenient, and made with synthetic color.

THE 1930s

Ivory skin with a waxy finish and a light touch of blush (if any) was the epitome of style in the 1930s. Makeup was sparse and lightly sun-kissed, with the blush applied like little roses on the "apples" of the cheeks.

To create this look, women reached for cream or powder blush. This was also when the idea that you could sculpt your face with the help of blush (depending on your face shape) gained momentum.

THE 1940s

Foundation and loose powder, applied with a swan's down puff, became an important part of 1940s makeup. To accentuate the look, blush was applied over the entire cheek and painted like an upside-down triangle. During the meager war years, women used a tried-and-true technique: simply pinching the skin to encourage healthy, rosy cheeks.

THE 1950s

Liquid foundation was very popular in the 1950s, as was powder and blush stored in handy cases. Brands like Elizabeth Arden, Max Factor, and Helena Rubinstein were a must in your handbag. For blush color, everyone was wearing pink. During this era, makeup was somewhat heavier than in previous decades, with the exception of blush.

Tip!

To avoid flecks on your cheek, tap the blush brush a little after swirling it in color. Circular motions result in a sweet and soft look, while sharp strokes yield a harder, tougher impression.

THE 1960s

The swinging '60s were mostly about the eyes and hair. Skin and lips were powdered. Blush was primarily used to shape the face. It was applied as a dash on the apples of the cheeks to emphasize the cheekbones. During this period, a new kind of blush, reminiscent of a large lipstick, was launched.

VINTAGE NAILS

Half moons, bare tips, and bright colors—
get creative with vintage-inspired nails!

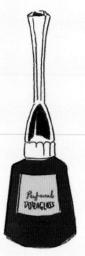

Nails in bright colors, inventive patterns, and creative shapes are no novelty. The fact is that trends have come and gone for thousands of years. To a large degree, painted nails have been a status symbol, a way to distinguish the upper class from the middle class.

Until the twentieth century, only the very rich could afford to paint their nails, but in time the advent of industrialization brought about affordable nail polish.

THE 1910s

According to the Edwardian fashion of the day, less was more. A high position in society was displayed through careful hygiene. Painted nails occured only in the highest levels of society, where the nails were "tinted" with pink or red oil. Modern nail polish was invented in 1917.

THE 1920s

Nail polish made a splash in the expressive fashion of the 1920s. Painting one's nails was considered rebellious, daring, and trendy. The colors were the same as the ones you'd see on modern cars: red, blue, and green. Almond-shaped nails were painted with bare tips. The half-moon manicure (see page 114) was another 1920s favorite.

𝒯ips!

• Use a base coat to minimize discoloration of the nail bed.

• Make sure each coat of polish is completely dry before applying the next.

• Invest in a quality topcoat to make sure your manicure lasts longer.

THE 1930s

Nail polish turned into a business. The world-famous makeup brand Revlon, which was founded in 1932, introduced its own nail polish (made with pigment). Hollywood was a main source of inspiration for the worlds of fashion and beauty. Whatever graced the silver screen soon made its way onto the pages of the stylish color magazines. Both the bare tip and the half-moon manicure stayed trendy in colors like pink and red and also appeared in more daring choices, such as emerald green.

THE 1940s

Lips were painted red and so were nails. To paint one's lips and nails in the exact same shade was sensational and a total novelty! Makeup brands introduced kits with matching lipstick and nail polish in shades of red and pink. Showing the half moon of the nail was still in fashion, but the trend was slowly but surely being chipped away at the edges.

THE 1950s

The whole nail painted in glorious Technicolor red—matched with red lips—was popular in the 1950s, along with the French manicure. Brand-new shimmering polishes in coral and pink were also introduced.

Color movies—such a spectacular innovation—inspired beauty and fashion. Anything seen on the movie stars quickly turned into a trend. In order to mimic the stars' polished perfection with their set hair, manicured round nails, and impeccable makeup, women headed to the beauty parlors. Showing that you could afford salon treatments was a status symbol in the 1950s.

THE 1960s

Pop-art nails, matching the graphic patterns and explosive colors in fashion, began to rival the classic red. Pastel green, yellow, lilac, and pink balanced the dark shades of the heavy eyeliner. Natural nails became increasingly popular with the younger crowd, who wished to take a step in the opposite direction of their primped parents' generation.

HALF-MOON MANICURE

When it comes to nails, the half-moon manicure is a real retro favorite. This style enjoyed immense popularity from the 1920s through the 1940s and has come back in vogue today.

You'll need

HOLE-PUNCH REINFORCEMENT OR
SCOTCH TAPE
SCISSORS
BASE COAT
COLORED COAT
TWEEZERS
TOPCOAT
COTTON SWAB
NAIL POLISH REMOVER

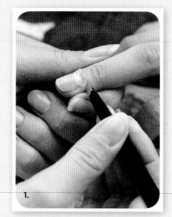

1.

1. Make your half-moon template by either cutting a hole-punch reinforcement in half or by cutting a piece of tape into a half circle. Apply a base coat to dry nails and wait for them to dry. Attach the half-moon template along the cuticle and press the template against the nail to make sure it sticks and is free from small creases where polish might accidentally sneak in.

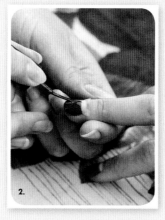

2.

2. Once the template is in place, apply the colored polish. Two coats is ideal. Make sure the first coat is completely dry before adding the next.

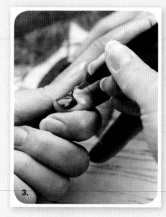

3.

3. Remove the template when the polish is semidry. If you wait too long, you risk removing polish in the process. Removing the stencil with your fingers can be a bit tricky, so tweezers can be helpful. Pull the template downward, in the direction of the finger, to avoid accidentally removing strips of polish.

4. Finish by applying a topcoat, so the edge left by the template gets a little extra coverage. Correct any mishaps with a cotton swab dipped in nail polish remover.

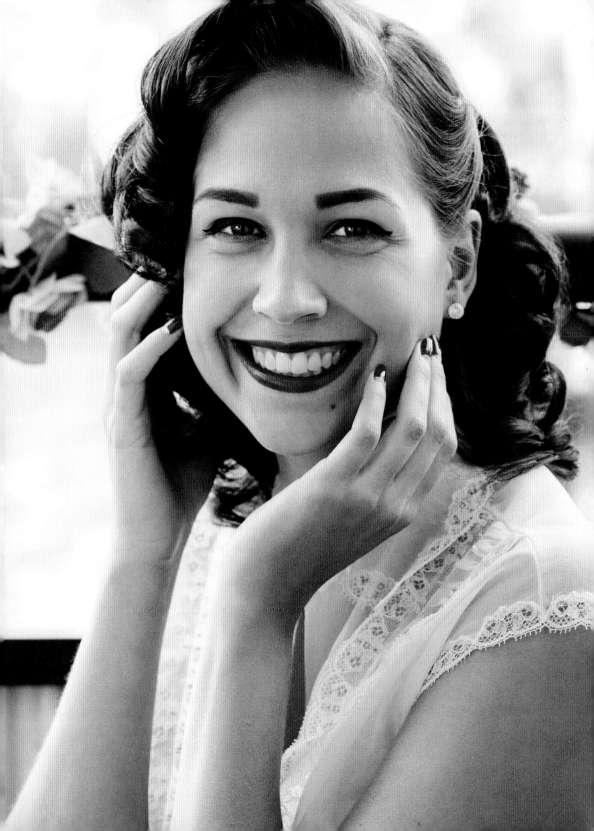

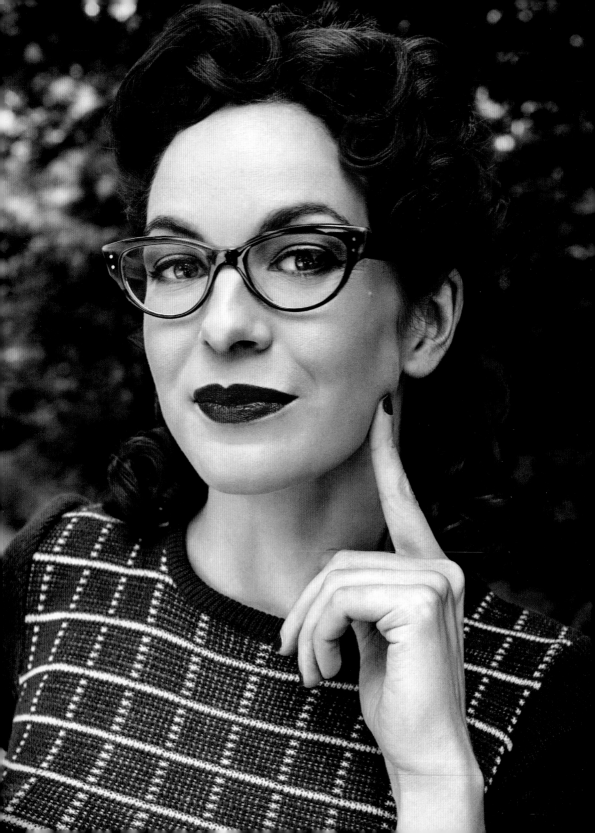

GLASSES

Glasses are distinctive, eye-catching, and a necessary evil.
This reluctant accessory has gone from understated to
iconic in just fifty years.

THE 1910s

The big question of this era was: Spectacles or a pince-nez (or even a monocle)? Round tortoiseshell frames were all the rage, paired with the puffed-up hair of the 1910s.

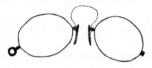

THE 1920s

During this period, function came before beauty. The glasses were round and unobtrusive to suit the precise, square bob cuts.

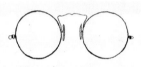

THE 1930s

As a number of hairstyle trends emerged—1930s curls, Veronica Lake waves, and short, set hairstyles—increasingly discreet glasses appeared on the market. The new sun-kissed trend brought about a new style of eyewear: sunglasses.

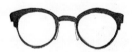

THE 1940s

"Scientific research" established that it was possible to beautify women with the help of glasses if one just stayed with the recommendations for each face shape. According to this theory, there were two face shapes: oval and round. Women with the round face shape should go for more angular glasses, while women with oval face shapes would look best in round glasses. For both face shapes, hairstyles that did not obscure the face were recommended. During the 1940s, glasses were made from metal, colored plastic, or both. It was during this period that brow-line glasses were launched—eyewear that was framed only on top.

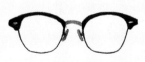

THE 1950s

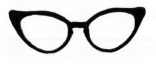

Eyewear became a fashion accessory in the '50s. Forget narrow, discreet metal glasses—bold frames took center stage. Horn-rimmed specs, brow-line models, and Ray-Ban Wayfarers were popular trends. But topping the blurred list were sharp, cat-eyed glasses worn with set curls and distinctive eyebrows (see page 109). Nothing got in the way of the angular, characteristic features. Another trend was decorated glasses. The cat-eyed glasses also came in glittering rhinestone versions—a must-have for any party.

THE 1960s

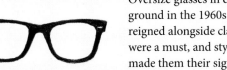

Oversize glasses in different shapes, colors, and patterns broke new ground in the 1960s. Narrow, elongated glasses with heavy frames reigned alongside classic Wayfarers and square models. Sunglasses were a must, and style icons like Jackie Kennedy and Brigitte Bardot made them their signature items alongside iconic hairstyles.

Psst!

A pair of eyeglasses can enhance a hairstyle in different ways. Cat-eyed models direct glances upward to a nice voluminous 'do. Thick horn-rimmed glasses emphasize distinct Bettie bangs. A sweet 'do can be made more daring and a daring 'do made sweeter with the help of different eyewear.

MAKEUP TRICKS FOR GIRLS WHO WEAR GLASSES

*Makeup and glasses are not always an easy
combination. Optimize your makeup
with these tips and tricks.*

1. When wearing glasses, use light-colored makeup around your eyes. A brightening concealer under the eye works wonders, as does a light eye shadow on your lids. Apply white eyeliner on the inside of the lower lid. This opens up the eye and compensates for any shadows caused by the glasses.

2. Double up! An extra dash of makeup helps your makeup show through the glasses. Be generous.

3. Here's a great rule of thumb: The thicker the frames, the more defined the lines need to be. Work with eyeliner, eyebrows, and lips to balance your bespectacled look.

Acknowledgments

Aurea Florio Fava
Linda Stålarm (Miss Stålarm)
Old Touch
TheMostestGirl
Peas & Understanding
The Flying Veterans
Citykonditoriet
Liljeholmsbadet
Chicago
Johan Ankarfyr
Betty the PV
Andreas Ridén
Maria Selinder
John Larsson
Helena Nilsson
Erica Olsson
Cristopher Overall

The Models:

Karoline Pettersson
Johanna Alm
Veronica Marino
Johanna Åkerblom
Cecilia Hedman
Ruby Luscious
Christina Morberg Segura
Sara Harjunen
Nanna Björnsson
Lina Östh
Liza Christensen
Kristin Harrysson
Linnea Levin
Alma Lindquist Anander
Emelie Eriksson
Julia Ortschütz

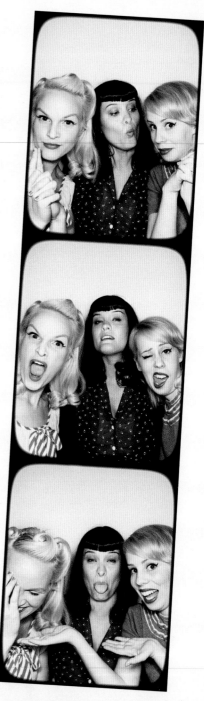

Sarah Wing is the renowned vintage hairstylist behind the Retroella salon. She has created hairstyle magic for a number of publications. She also arranges popular classes on vintage hairstyling at her own vintage-styled salon in Stockholm.

Emma Sundh is a freelance journalist (specializing in contemporary history), a vintage blogger (emmasvintage.se), and an illustrator. She has worked in magazines for the past seven years, most recently at *Damernas Värld.* The most popular topic on her blog? Hairstyles, hairstyles, and hairstyles.

Martina Ankarfyr is a photographer whose elegant pictures are the perfect match for this book's vintage theme. She is also the photographer behind books such as *Vintageparty, Pärlans konfektyr,* and *StikkiNikki Icepops.*

First published in the United States of America in 2015
by Chronicle Books LLC.

First published in Sweden in 2014 by Norstedts as
Vintage frisyrer.

Library of Congress Cataloging-in-Publication Data:
Sundh, Emma.
   Vintage hairstyles : simple steps for retro hair with a
   modern twist
   / Emma Sundh, Sarah Wing ; photographs by Martina
Ankarfyr.
    pages cm
   ISBN 978-1-4521-4308-8
   1. Hairstyles. I. Wing, Sarah. II. Title.

TT972.S795 2014
646.7'24—dc23

                                        2014049156

Manufactured in China

Design and layout: Katy Kimbell
All photography: Martina Ankarfyr
Illustrations: Emma Sundh
Prepress: Elanders Fälth & Hässler, Värnamo
English translation by Emi Guner

10 9 8 7 6 5 4 3 2

Chronicle Books LLC
680 Second Street
San Francisco, California 94107
www.chroniclebooks.com